TREADSIDE MANNER

CONFESSIONS OF A SERIAL PERSONAL TRAINER

By Greg Justice

ISBN-10: 1470111535
ISBN-13: 978-1470111533

The author disclaims responsibility or adverse effects or consequences from the misapplication or injudicious use of the information contained in this book. Mention of resources and associations does not imply an endorsement.

Design: Nancy McDonald

fit-pro.com
FB.com/greg.justice1
Twitter.com/aycfit
GregJustice@aycfit.com

To my wife, Dana,
children, David, Kale and Mia,
and my brother Jeff

1. Don't Burn Bridges

- Treadside Manner:
    - Dress / Carry yourself
    - Way you act/react *Think
    - Enthusiastically Introducing your product
    - Your Expertise in Exercise Science + Progression
        * Before you think outside the box... learn what's inside the box.
    - Your Support & Motivational Guidance
    - You Guarantee of Success (2 way Street)

5 P's Purpose, Passion, Persuasion, Perseverance, + Patience

Relationship Ladder
- Educate -
- Interrigation

Hearing, Listening, Purposeful Listening

Topics to advoid w/ Clients
- Political   Its their session
- Religion
- Gossip (move on next set)

Goals vs. Dreams
Example: loose 40lbs vs. She wants to fit in her little red dress she first met her husband

Personal and Profesinal

CONTENTS

ACKNOWLEDGMENTS

During the past thirty years I have been blessed to come in contact with so many people and organizations that have helped me along the way and inspired this book. To each and every one of them I am truly grateful, for it has been their support and inspiration that has enabled me to make this book a reality.

First, I would like to thank my wife, Dana. Without her love, patience and support this book would not exist. Next, my children, David, Kale and Mia, who, along with my wife, inspire me to do what I do.

Many other individuals deserve thanks for assisting and inspiring me along the way. Thanks to all of my trainers, past and present. I am especially grateful to Glen Haney (AYC manager since 1994) and Nadine Price-Rojas (AYC Yoga instructor since 1994) for their long time support and dedication to AYC; Current staff, Ellen Breeding, Sean Dill, Marci Farrar, Katie Kinkaid-Longhauser, Nancy Levin, Nancy McDonald, Derek Newman, and Stephanie Switzer; Former AYC trainers, Tim Johnson, Darin Fletcher and Ryan Layman; and Mary Bartnik, Amy Hicks, and Nancy McDonald for helping me put these stories on paper and editing.

Thank you to all of my clients, past and present, including Jeanne Olofson for inspiring the term "Treadmill Topics" and being an advocate and supporter of AYC Health & Fitness, and me, for nearly a quarter of a century; My 'Core 20', Dave Seitter, Harold and Ruthie Tivol, Alan and Joan Marsh, Addie Ward, Julia Kauffman, Barbara Seidlitz, Tom and Jeanne Olofson, Dick and Sandy Berkley,

Debbie Ward, Barbara Marshall, Laura Welch, Annette Bloch, John Mueller, Myron and Nikki Wang, and David Stickelber.

Thanks also to the following individuals and organizations: Fitness Consulting Group (Pat Rigsby and Nick Berry), NPE (Sean Greeley, Eric Ruth, Dick Chilton and Camelia Herndon), Fitness Branding 101 (Rocco Castellano), Kick Back Life (Chris McCombs), SuperTrainer.com (Sam Bakhtiar and Kaiser Serajuddin), Boot Camp Automator (BJ Gaddour), Fitness Business Interviews (Erik Rokeach), Jim Labadie, PFP (Personal Fitness Professional magazine), IDEA (Health & Fitness Association), and AFAA (Aerobics and Fitness Association of America).

And finally, a very special thank you to Dax Moy for agreeing to do the forward for this book and being an inspiration to our industry. You are the best Dax Moy I've ever met, even though I'll never meet that Dax Moy again. Thank you, my friend.

FOREWORD
BY DAX MOY

There aren't many individuals within the personal training profession that I'd write a personal foreword to their book for yet when Greg asked me to put together an introduction to his latest creation I eagerly jumped at the opportunity.

Why?

Quite simply, Greg is one of the most experienced trainers in the world, having clocked up tens of thousands of client contact hours over more than 30 years in-the-trenches as a fitness professional, and during this time has managed to maintain an open mind and an open heart to new ideas, concepts, and practices as they brush up against this adolescent industry of ours.

Better yet, he's managed to remain a thoughtful, humble, and generous individual who's still passionately in love with what he does and those he does it for which, in an industry of increasing cynicism, sets him apart from fully 99% of trainers who often fall more in love with the marketing practices associated with being a trainer than with being a trainer itself.

Lest you think this is some 'old boys network' backslapping going on here, I must admit to only having met Greg face to face for the first time about 6 weeks ago and before then only ever having known him through

Facebook and online communities. We've never done the 'my good friend' cross referrals and affiliate-thing so common among strangers these days, and have never gained financially from exposing a single product to our 'lists' either (I always wonder why we call our tribal communities 'lists' and de-personalize them when we are supposed to be about 'personal' training).

Yet despite our personal acquaintance only having been made recently, I feel a deep abiding respect and trust for the man who I've seen share of himself so selflessly and consistently over the past 5 years I've watched him online. (Yes Greg, I've watched you!) :)

That's why I'm really pleased to be part of his latest offerings to help the profession to remember (or to recognize for the first time) the amazingly important and powerful role we play with our clients and how it's often the small things (which really aren't that small) that tend to make the biggest impact on the lives we touch during the course of our working lives.

Greg shares the teachings of literally decades of experience through a series of reflections on conversations that have often occurred during the treadmill warm-up portion of his training sessions, an often overlooked element by junior trainers, and reveals not-so-secret secrets, strategies, skills and the 'special sauce' that has created client retention that averages 20 years and more.

I urge you to read Greg's stories. Not just some, but all, as buried within the lines of each one is a prescription for making both a great living and a great difference in what is arguably the most important profession in the world.

Being a trainer is easy these days. A weekend certification and you're well on your way to earning a decent living. Yet being a GREAT trainer is, as my nan used to say 'a different kettle of fish' (I think Greg may have taught her that when she was a little girl... Just joking Greg!) and is a mix of both art and science. This may not be a science-based book, but the art that Greg shares will dramatically transform your career... if you apply it.

Truth, joy and love,

Dax Moy
The UK's Leading Personal Training Coach
Author Of 'The MAGIC Hundred Goal Achievement Program"

INTRODUCTION

It's hard to believe that 30 years have passed since I entered this industry and the truth is, I feel like I've only just begun.

I am truly blessed to do what I love to do, everyday.

During the past 30 years, I have worked with hundreds of fitness professionals and helped them gain a better understanding of what makes a great personal trainer. My mission is to do everything I can to elevate the professional and ethical standards of an industry for which I have great passion. Without passion for what you do, you simply cannot reach, or sustain a level of excellence that our industry needs and deserves.

Personal training is both an art and a science. While both are equally important, in this book, I chose to focus on the 'art' of personal fitness training. Too many times, the art of personal training is forgotten. I know lots of smart, well educated trainers that are broke because they can't relate to their clients. They don't truly listen to what's being said. They're too set in their ways to deviate from a certain one-size-fits-all game plan to know what their client(s) really need.

In this book, I write about:

- What motivates an individual to hire a personal trainer?
- What makes them stay with a certain trainer for long periods of time?

- How *really* listening to your clients can help you grow your business.
- What topics are safe to discuss with your clients and which ones you should avoid.
- How to overcome obstacles.
- Simple ways to over-deliver to your clients.
- A few trends during the past 30 years
- A tribute to the "godfather of fitness", Jack LaLanne.

The stories in this book are real and they've helped define who I am as a Christian, husband, father, friend, and businessman. I hope they will inspire you to be the best personal trainer you can be.

And one last thing…I can truly say that my joy and passion for this industry is as strong today as it was the day I began more that 30 years ago, and I wish for you the same joy and passion.

God Bless,
Greg Justice

TREADSIDE MANNER

CONFESSIONS OF A SERIAL PERSONAL TRAINER

1

YOUR TREADSIDE MANNER
IS PART OF YOUR PRODUCT

Do you remember the very first product you ever offered to your prospects and clients? Think back long, long ago when you were first starting out.

Your first product was *time with you*, the trainer who would provide an excellent experience and proven results in record time.

You packaged yourself in how you dressed and carried yourself. You enthusiastically introduced the components of your product one by one, your expertise in exercise progression, your supportive motivational elements, and your guidance needed to reach their goals. You used your environment to help set the stage for this great product, you offered a guarantee with your product, and you priced out your product accordingly.

Prospects became clients when they liked the look and the promise of the product they were buying. And if you, the product, delivered as stated, most of them continued to purchase more time with you, the Trainer.

If, on the other hand, many of them did not renew their time with you, what did you do? Did you go back to the drawing board to recreate your product? Or perhaps you added some 'special features' like discounts, additional assessments, or maybe a free pedometer or nutrition/exercise record log.

Take a look back at your original product, and take a look now, compare them.

Back then were you so determined to help people that your care and concern shone forth ever so brightly in your excellent treadside manner? Back then did you individualize each client so they felt they were your favorite client and they basked in the attention and love they got from you?

Your treadside manner is what sells your product, you, time after time. That treadside manner is what your clients tell others about, it's the reason they love you and stay with you. It's the largest component of the product you offer.

In the way that some patients prefer a doctor who is all business and others prefer a doctor who will hold their hand, so too it goes with Personal Trainers.

Do you have an innate sense of what each person wants or needs to carry on, to commit, to succeed? If not, simply ask them, and then deliver it.

Today, right now, how many of your clients tell other people, "I know I'm one of Greg's favorite clients"? Or favorite groups, or favorite classes? Those are the clients that love your treadside manner and have connected with you through it.

If your treadside manner is adaptable to individual desires, if you mirror them, and give them what they need as individuals, you will renew the majority of your clients, no matter how diverse.

Does your current treadside manner shine forth with individualized attention that balances your client preferences in the relationship and the business of training?

Don't know? Ask some of your favorite clients if they realize they are your favorite client then listen and watch for their response. It just may make your day!

2

LISTEN WITH A PURPOSE

At any given point during the day or night you can enter your gym and be greeted by familiar sounds of clanging equipment, straining clients, encouraging trainers, the news channel, music and a hubbub of voices mixed in. The familiarity of all these sounds is comforting to your subconscious when you are on track with your goals and want to be there. That same familiarity of sounds is not comforting when you are stressed, not on track, and don't want to be there at that particular time.

We HEAR familiar sounds passively. They just happen and enter our ears. It is our choice if they go further into our conscious level. That choice to let the sounds in is called LISTENING. Listening is active.

Have you ever been in your gym and the familiar sounds have been in the background of your mind without you paying attention when all of a sudden there is a larger, deep thud that you don't normally hear and all the background noise and voices stop instantly so all you hear is the news channel? In that split second the unfamiliarity of sounds raised an alarm in your brain and you got right into action to not only listen, but to see and investigate what happened.

You knew it probably wasn't a good thing.

Sometimes it takes a shift in sounds to get our attention. Sometimes we are so pre-occupied with other things that we are not paying attention to something that we should. Other than our business itself, the most important thing we should be paying attention to is our clients. They pay our bills and give us our livelihood. They help us build our business when we pay attention to them, when we really listen to them. They can tear it down when they feel we aren't listening to them, their needs, their concerns.

Purposeful listening while you have your client on the treadmill can really open your eyes to possibilities and opportunities. It can also help you detect potential problems, build rapport, and create a trusting relationship that is so important to people before they open up and reveal very much about themselves or their lives.

There is also a big difference between listening and purposeful listening. When you listen you can answer a question or return a comment. With purposeful listening you can delve deeper into a topic that will lead to a more productive dialogue, a stronger relationship, and more profit in your business.

Purposeful listening has gotten me leads to many of my clients and many corporate accounts, too. Purposeful listening is how I've been able to keep many of my clients more than 10, 15, and 20 years, helping me grow my business and enrich my life.

Now, go meet with your next client and ask them a purposeful question and really listen. It will lead somewhere good when you listen purposefully.

3

LISTENING TO YOUR INVESTMENT

"It was like breaking up with a girlfriend." - When one of my trainers came to me with this statement, I heard and saw his frustration with a client who said, "You're a great trainer, but..."

This client/trainer relationship had been a three year 'hearing but not listening' tug of war as the client denied and refused to stop certain lifestyle behaviors outside of the gym that were thwarting the efforts of trainer and client in the gym.

Trust and communication between trainer and client are central to setting and achieving goals and fulfilling the vision. A few minutes at a time, a few days each week, they communicate their very life to you, creating a bond of friendship, trust, and mutual work (or play).

Your client/trainer relationships are investments you make in your business.

Sometimes those relationships stay strong and continue to grow year after year. Sometimes they deteriorate, or never get off the ground from the start. Some are a combination of ups and downs, with a few twists mixed in.

Listen and you can hear what is important to them. Listen between the lines and you'll hear what makes them tick. "Listen" to their facial expressions, their body language, and their choice of words as they respond to their latest measurement or assessment results. That moment is a window of opportunity to grow that relationship investment to new heights.

Listen and watch. You may see and hear joy and a sense of accomplishment, jubilance; one of the moments every personal trainer lives for. This is the client we all want, the one whose accountability produces the work, results, and achievement.

If you see dread in their eyes, hear excuses coming from their mouth, defeat in the sag of their body, they are speaking to you loud and clear. There are some obstacles in their life, in their habits, in their thinking. Some have unsupportive family members, some have deep seeded emotional eating issues, and some are party animals outside the gym. These people who have sabotage in their daily life will not achieve their goals unless they face that obstacle and make some determined and definite change.

This is the point where you, as their trainer, must step up your communication with them. Ask them the difficult questions and don't settle for evasive answers. Acknowledge their struggle and help them find the determination to overcome those obstacles and rise to the next level. Otherwise, you've lost that client even if they continue working out with you.

By filling a time slot and going through the motions, that relationship is no longer built on trust and real goals. If you continue to "train" them, you have "settled" for an unfulfilling trainer/client relationship that can hinder your growth.

Listen well to your investment with your ears, your eyes, and your heart. Don't settle for an unfulfilling trainer/client relationship, because your business will only grow in the direction you grow.

4

TREADMILL TOPICS TO EMBRACE AND AVOID

Toastmasters offers an impromptu opportunity at their meetings called Table Topics. Saturday Night Live had a segment they called Coffee Talk. I have what I call Treadmill Topics. This is my opportunity to build a strong relationship with my clients. As they warm up on the treadmill we have conversation and I can learn a lot about them, and share some about me. We strengthen our bond as we work toward achieving their goals. I am also finding out how I can serve them better, whom they know that I can get a referral to, and opportunities to keep strengthening that bond.

Here are some Quick Silver Topics (money in your pocket) I use:

Profession/Work Life
- Where they work
- What they do
- What they find most interesting about what they do
- What they find most challenging about what they do
- If they could do anything, would they still do what they are doing?
- How long have they done that?
- How long have they been there?
- Who to contact for a corporate fitness program, if they don't have one

- How their corporate fitness program is going, if they have one - if it's working, why are they with you?
- Their dreams for their future

Summary: If they are looking to grow, get promoted, change occupations, etc. you may know something you can share - a contact, an opportunity, an opening, etc. If you are looking to grow, they may know something they will share with you - a contact, referral, recommendation, working knowledge of a corporate process, etc.

Family/Home Life
- Children
- Spouse
- Pets
- Food they eat, times they eat
- What makes their family special?
- Kids schooling
- Kid's future schooling/military, etc.
- Their dreams for their family's future

Summary: A person's family, especially kids, is often a source of joy and pride (yes, headaches and worries, too). Share those joys (and headaches) with them; you will be strengthening your relationship with them.

Social/Activity Life
- Hobbies
- Individual activities
- Group activities
- Church
- Alma mater, alumni?
- Sports
- Personal best/weekend warrior

Summary: These are usually fun and interesting times for your clients. They belong to something larger than themselves, they challenge themselves through these activities, or they just plain enjoy them. Share that joy with them and you may find yourself with another whole group for boot camp.

In the course of doing business, the most important element is the human element. Relationship and communication will help you keep them as clients and make them ready, willing, and able to provide you with other prospects. Don't overlook the opportunities for growth in your own business that your current clients can help provide to you. Use my Treadmill Topics and develop some of your own and watch your prospect list and your business grow.

Here are some Quick Sand Topics I NEVER use (engulfed in controversy):

- Religion
- Sex & Extra Marital Affairs
- Gossip
- Politics
- Other Clients
- Crossing Professional Boundaries
- Any Topic where your client has obvious extreme views one way or another
- Personal issues*

*Double Quick Sand Topic to never, ever use:

- Never bring your hardships, complaints, problems, or any kind of personal issue into the working relationship. It's one thing to share a tidbit of how you overcame something that your client is facing at the current time.

It is inappropriate and unprofessional to bring your personal issues before a client. It's also a big turn-off and you risk losing that client as well as any prospects they may have recommended.

Summary: In any business you want to build strong relationships that help promote and nurture the bond that keeps your clients coming back. It's not only the results you give them, it's also your "bedside manner", your personality, your willingness to give them that little extra attention...All relationships have the potential for disaster. If you stay away from these topics and stick with the ones listed in the Quick Silver section, you will be building strong bonds that will help grow your business. You will be able to get more referrals and leads from your clients because they find you caring, trustworthy, and respectful, as well as knowledgeable. Stay away from controversy. Stick with the topics near and dear to their heart, and relevant to their life. It is all about them.

5

FINE TUNED FOCUS HELPS YOU FIND MORE TIME

Much like you, I run boot camps, do personal and small group training, corporate boot camps and wellness programs, run a number of businesses, speak, write, and still have the endless communications to deal with in addition to staying up on the industry research, trends, and discoveries.

And I have a family and a social life.

One thing I did that helped me in a very big way was to *focus on one thing*. Not wanting any aspect of my business to suffer, I found the common denominator and created the focus from there.

My focus: health & fitness.

My message: Without regular exercise and proper nutrition, the body will begin to deteriorate into a state of disease.

My menu of services: The same as before.

My marketing: All geared toward the benefits of health and fitness. Yes, some products and classes have more marketing copy that is geared specifically to that product or class, yet they all start with health and fitness. That is the bottom line.

So, what I did was clearly identify the focus of my business as creating health and fitness in everyone. That way, no matter who I am talking with (in business), the subject is always health & fitness as I assess their needs and desires, then steer them in the direction of the product/service that suits them best.

What changed?

My brain focus.
My clarity of thinking.
My purpose.

The speed with which my brain is tuned into the conversation or response is fantastic. I can pull in examples from any type of class or session for anyone I am talking to and match the benefits the prospect is looking for.

The reality is that if you chunk down regular exercise and proper nutrition far enough, you wind up with health and fitness. Yes, you get a toned and/or muscular body, you get greater balance, agility, and flexibility, but you also get health benefits, a greater quality of life, and longevity.

6

"AND THEY'RE WILLING TO PAY YOU FOR THAT?"

Once upon a time, you had a dream.

Did someone help you to nurture that dream and help you see it become reality?

Whether you had that encouraging force in your life or not, you can look back and see the fervor, the desire, the obstacles, the fear, the pain, and the driving force it took you to get there.

You built another dream on top of that one, didn't you?

With each achievement we set our sights higher and higher. Sometimes with each obstacle we let our dreams fall by the wayside. The path to the Holy Grail is littered with broken and discarded dreams. Those dreams once held the deepest desires, fondest wishes, and the very heartbeat of the dreamer.

Back in the early to mid 80's personal training wasn't like it is now. When I told my wife about my dreams of starting a personal training business, her response was, "and they're willing to pay you for that?" She couldn't comprehend the idea of an individual paying someone to do a workout in a one-on-one setting and paying a fee.

Though she didn't understand, she helped by encouraging and nurturing my dream into reality.

Your clients are more likely to express a goal to you. They are less likely to share a dream with you unless they sense that you genuinely care about them. They will sense your care and support when you actively listen to them are focused on them and are avoiding distractions.

The goal is a 40 lb. weight loss. The dream that spurs that goal is the little black dress in the back of the closet and the thought of dancing in the arms of her husband once again.

The goal is to get stronger and bulk up. The dream may be to stand tall and get out from under that bully once and for all.

The goal is to achieve maximum health. The dream may really be the fear of becoming disabled and suffering a slow, painful death like a parent did.

What are your clients paying you for? Personal training? That's what the contract says. Yet, in their hearts, they have hired you to help nurture their dreams into the reality they want so strongly that they can taste it.

"If all your workout goals were achieved and became reality overnight, when you wake up tomorrow morning, what would your life look like?" "What will your life look like when you achieve those workout goals?" Ask them, listen to what they have to say, and then nurture their dreams into reality.

Dreams are just as precious today as they were back in the mid 80's. Handle them with care. They are the roadmap to success in client retention. They are a stepping stone for you to traverse with your client in building a deeper, richer relationship that will not only help them achieve their dreams, but also to help you achieve yours along the way.

7

HAVE YOU HAD YOUR SALLY FIELD MOMENT?

If your clients are happy, and they like what you're doing for them, they will keep coming back. Client retention equals cash flow. If you don't have good retention rates, interview your clients. Find out what they are thinking.

I interviewed a group of clients I call my "core 20" and I asked them three simple questions;

1. What was your original motivation for hiring a personal fitness trainer?

2. Why did you choose Greg Justice to be your trainer?

3. Why have you chosen to stay with one trainer for so long? (All of them 15+ years.)

Here is a summary of what my "Core 20" told me...

They originally hired a personal fitness trainer to get healthy, gain strength and endurance and benefit from one-on-one attention. There's nothing too surprising there, just straight forward and to the point.

Why me?

Here's where my hard work really started to pay off. Nearly every one of them said someone else personally referred them to me, and that my reputation as a personal trainer is what motivated them to call me. We've all heard that word of mouth is a personal trainer's best form of advertising, and this really confirmed that for me. Never underestimate the power of personal referrals.

Why have they stayed with one trainer so long? Okay, this is where my head begins to swell, but just a little. An interesting theme developed, every single survey came back with at least one sentence that mentioned that I was very easy to get along with, and that they enjoyed being around me. A few years ago an actress, named Sally Field, accepted her Oscar by saying "You like me, you really like me!" This was my "Sally Field" moment.

The second most common theme was that I never brought my personal issues into their session, but was always willing to concentrate on theirs.

Thirdly, was the ability to adapt as each session brought a new challenge; a sore neck or back; or they're tired, or stressed out because of personal reasons. Whatever the reason, you must be able to adapt every session to what's going on with your client that day.

There were a few mentions of my advanced degrees, my experience, reliability and dedication. I was called a "consummate professional" and "a joy!" While all of that was very flattering, it made me take a close look at what was important to my clients.

What's important to your clients? They want to like you and to know that your focus is on them. They want each session personalized just for them. If a client likes you, they will like your facility. If they don't like you, then no matter how nice your studio is or how many degrees and certifications you have--they won't like it, and they won't stay.

Interview your "core 20" clients today and maybe you'll have a Sally Field moment, too!

8

"IF IFS AND BUTS WERE CANDY AND NUTS... OH WHAT A PARTY WE COULD HAVE"

Creating a motivating momentum that will squash the 'ifs' and 'buts' can be very effective in client retention when you tackle it from two fronts simultaneously.

How?

By cementing their long term and short-term goals clearly identified in their minds with benefits vividly painted AND providing the spice and variety of challenges, achievements, and recognition in their sessions with you.

As Trainers, we've heard just about all the excuses in the book and then some as to why clients aren't achieving the success they want and why they can't or won't continue their sessions. Unfortunately, it's human nature to find the path of least resistance and to fall back into our comfort ruts.

Once a client has stopped coming to class and we look back over the conversations of the past months, we can see a progression of subtle hints disguised as jokes, overflowing responsibility, and even doubts. If we haven't helped address those statements and cement the client's commitment to exercise, it will be no surprise that they don't follow through for the long haul.

When they have both, the long range and short term cemented in their minds, that commitment will follow through in their actions. It will be easier to call them on self-sabotaging dialogue you hear from them.

The balance of mind/body/spirit will all come into play in our actions, thoughts, and words. When we listen to a client telling us the reason they will miss the next session, we can assess how they have balanced the importance of that event with the importance and value of their regular exercise sessions.

We can hear how their priorities are coming into focus. Each communication is an opportunity to help them align their goals, both long term and short term with their priorities.

We all have unavoidable events that crop up in our lives and unexpected visits or surprises that we want to take advantage of, causing us to rework our schedules. These are generally the exceptions that will not prevent our clients from staying focused on their goals. They are the spice and variety of life that helps us to renew and invigorate our commitment and focus.

In both personal training sessions and boot camps, change them up regularly to keep the spice and variety alive for your clients. Challenge them and recognize their accomplishments to help create a motivating momentum.

When you reinforce and cement the goals, they drop into the background as a fact of their life and they turn their focus to the enjoyment and work of the session at hand.

Listen to the 'ifs' and 'buts' your clients express.

Are their goals cemented?

Can they see, taste, and feel them?

Are you providing your clients with enough spice and variety, challenge and recognition that they need to offset the importance and value of their 'ifs' and 'buts'?

You didn't just say 'but' did you?

9

IT'S ALL ABOUT THEM
(SO IT CAN BE ALL ABOUT YOU IN THE LONG RUN)

When you make your sessions all about your client and really listen to them, you are empowering them to disclose things they hold close. They will reveal their desires, needs, fears, passions, hopes and dreams, and so much more. Treat those things they disclose with care and concern, respect and privacy.

You will discover things that hold clues to what may be hindering your client or putting them at risk of dropping out.

You can address those things and nip them in the bud by first acknowledging them and then helping the client work through them. You'll keep your clients a lot longer when they feel that it's all about them.

If they are feeling it, that is their reality. Do not dismiss their feelings, their reality. Help them to see the big picture, the greater reality, yet be supportive of what they are feeling.

Find that balance. Dig in deeper with them.

Listen for the main point your client is trying to get across.

When you develop your listening skills and bring them to play in every interaction with your clients, it changes the dynamics of the relationship. They work harder for you knowing that you really know them and care about them. They know this because they have heard it and seen it in the way you interact with them. They share more with you. Their sessions get livelier and they have more fun.

Here are some tips to practice that will help you listen well…

- Maintain eye contact.

- Don't interrupt.

- Stay still.

- Nod your head when you understand or agree.

- Lean in occasionally.

These body language skills show them that you are really paying attention to them. It is encouragement to them to keep talking and dig in deeper. People who feel appreciated and understood tend to be happier people and have an easier time overcoming obstacles through discussion. They also become very good clients who often bring in more clients.

When you use these skills, then pull out their main point and repeat it back to them in your own words, they know (and so do you) that you were really listening and that you understand what they were saying.

Sometimes it is not relevant whether you agree or disagree. Sometimes they just need to feel heard.

If they are talking too much, it will be easier to keep them on track with their program with a gentle nudge because they feel satisfied their message was heard. Often they will experience a sense of renewed vigor at being understood.

Practice these skills with the next person you see - client or not. Experience the difference good listening skills make in a conversation and in your grasp of it.

Use these skills and with each and every client you have and they will *know* that you know it's all about them.

10

I THOUGHT YOU MEANT…

George Bernard Shaw once said, "The single biggest problem in communication is the illusion that it has taken place."

Ever have a discussion with a client where both of you unknowingly walk away with a different understanding of what you both discussed?

Usually you find out later, during another discussion that sounds something like, "…Oh, I thought you meant (fill in the blank)". You think one thing while the other person is thinking something quite different, yet you are both under the illusion you communicated about the same thing.

Sometimes it's a simple miscommunication such as the time I sent an email late at night asking for a meeting "tomorrow". The following morning I received a confirmation of the meeting and at the appointed time she did not show up. I found out later that day that she opened the email in the morning and didn't look at the date of the email, assuming the word "tomorrow" meant the following day.

I made a mental note and set up my own policy of using the day or date instead of "tomorrow". Another example is the use of time zones when dealing with people around the country. We can communicate with people nationally or globally as though they were in the next room and forget that their 2 p.m. is different than our 2 p.m.

Imagine thinking that you clearly understand a message and you forge ahead with confidence, only to find out later that the time, alternate scheduling, money, and effort you put into it was wasted, or worse yet, created a set-back. It's happened to all of us.

One very simple and effective way to combat miscommunication is to repeat back what you think you heard in your own words. Summarizing the key action points of your communications goes a long way to creating effective communication and placing everyone involved on the same page

There are many other ways to beef up your communication to ensure that it is correctly understood. Putting it in writing is very effective, as long as it is clear. Signage, newsletters, and bulletin board posts all reinforce your message and provide additional confirmation with accuracy.

Consistency in communication is another. When the messages you write and the ones you speak are consistent, people are more in tune with your communications.

The best and most effective method to ensure accurate communications is to have systems in place for all aspects of your fitness business. Written systems for scheduling, payments, hiring, referrals, scripting, lead generation, closing the contracts, even the procedures for opening and closing your studio each day save time, money and misunderstanding.

Married couples that finish each other's sentences, staff that confidently proceed to the next step, clients who are comfortable and know what to expect...these are all products of consistent and accurate communication.

When people assume or fill in the blanks themselves, their assumptions are only as good as the information they have. Sometimes you only get one shot. Make it an effective one with excellent communication.

11

WHAT ISN'T BEING SAID

The client who shows up religiously for their exercise program, brings in their completed meal/water/exercise logs, asks questions, and tracks their progress in relation to the goals they worked out with you is the dream client who communicates well and seems most likely to get the best results from their program with you, one would think.

We've all had the clients who tell us what they 'want' and we work with them digging into their needs and desires to put together a fabulous plan that includes all the best in exercise and nutrition mixed in with healthy lifestyle choices.

Laboring with due diligence and care to keep them progressing, what happens when 3 weeks, 4 weeks down the road something is obviously amiss? We ask them questions to uncover the source of why things aren't going according to plan. Minor changes are made based on what they tell you, yet 5 weeks, 6 weeks, 7 weeks into their program something is still amiss.

What is it that they are NOT telling you?

Some things clients might NOT be saying:

• What their main objective really is and why they are taking your program.

- Who they are exercising for. Are they just trying to please someone else to say they did it?
- What they use as a measure and definition of results. You think body fat %, they think weight.
- They don't understand what you are saying and don't want to look 'dumb' so they won't ask.
- What they really think of you and your program.
- What's really happening with their body, mind, and spirit, and how it is affecting their daily life choices and their plan of action in achieving their goals.
- They think they found a better way but won't tell you, they just quit your program.
- They have pain and won't speak up or deny having the pain when you notice diminished movement.

Sometimes our clients honestly don't realize that they are living at cross purposes to their stated goals and other times they know and are simply hoping things will still work out for them. We need to look for clues in other areas of our conversations with them to help the communication process.

Take the case of one client who was keeping faithful food logs, exercising with me three times each week and yet couldn't lose a single pound over many months (body fat % stayed about the same too). After telling me about a margarita lunch at work, I finally put it all together. She didn't equate 3 or 4 margarita lunches each week with any extra calories, sugar, or carbs in her diet, nor did it click with the beer she consumed on the weekends. In her mind, they didn't count.

For some clients, keeping them on track, keeping them as clients longer, and keeping them happy to refer you to their friends takes a bit of digging to find out what isn't being said.

Start digging today!

12

MAKE IT PERSONAL, KEEP IT PROFESSIONAL

One of my long-time clients recently said, "You make it personal while always keeping it professional."

She said that upon completing her 3,168th personal training session with me. She's one of 20 personal training clients that have been with me for more than 20 years...you do the math on 'life-time' value of clients like that.

What is it that creates and sustains a 20-year trainer/client relationship in an industry with only a 31% client retention average longer than 5 years? How does a trainer achieve greater than average client retention?

You create a special world just for them, a world they will want to visit 3,168 times and counting. They will carve out a small chunk of their time to visit a world that was made just for them, for their benefit, structured with their values and preferences.

Make it Personal, Keep it Professional simply means do your job well for each and every client as if they were your only client.

We live in a day and age where many people feel lack of control over most areas of their time and life, where responsibilities and commitments can sometimes be overwhelming.

Some people appreciate a time and space where they can go to 'breathe'. Others want expert guidance to help them stay the course. Some understand the value of exercise in relation to their health and well-being. Almost all of them will feel the benefits of exercise faster when their trainer hears what they want and provides it.

The world you create for them, on their terms will offer an environment that is enriching and nurturing to them. Some thrive on a high energy, fast paced group, while others embrace the privacy of one-on-one. Some want to work only on equipment and can't shake their old school roots. Others want to be challenged continually; some need constant confirmation of their progress.

When you listen to your clients, you can easily create a world with them at the center. As they voice their perspectives on a variety of topics, you can hear their values and boundaries, their likes and dislikes, their favorites, their opinions, and what makes them tick.

The world you create for each client will be a little bit different. If we try to fit them all into the same mold many of them won't fit, won't be happy, and won't come back.

Listen for their preferences and create that special world, just for them – even if it's a large group boot camp, you can still help them glow in their own special place with a bit of attention, a well placed wink or nod, a few words of their accomplishments, acknowledgement that you know they are working hard and are proud of them. Show them you hear them, see them, and value them.

Personal and Professional....together in one sentence is the ultimate ideal world for a client in the fitness setting. That perfect combination makes a world of difference to a client and a trainer working toward the future together.

13

BRIDGES ARE MADE FOR CROSSING, NOT BURNING

Building strong, lasting professional relationships during your career is something that you should research, begin immediately, and continue throughout your career. A reputation for professionalism, honesty, and competence can be determined by your activities at just one job.

In the early 80's, I was managing a workout center when it was sold. As soon as the new owners came in, they completely "cleaned house". They fired the entire management team – which included me. Instead of reacting negatively, telling them that they didn't know what they were doing, or venting my anger, I stayed calm, remained professional, and commanded the respect of the owners due to my reaction.

Then, devastated, I went home to tell my wife of six months that I had been fired. This was one of the hardest things I have ever had to do. Clearly, my personal situation and my communication with the owners should not have – and did not – exhibit the same characteristics. Personal feelings should not impact your professional conduct with your employer, even if you are being terminated. Complete disassociation is, of course, impossible, but the greater the separation of the two, the more capable you will appear.

Two days later the new owner called to offer my job back, because a lot of the members complained that I was no longer there. Since I had already made plans to finish my master's degree out of state, I made him an offer. I said that I would come back to work there in 5 months, after I completed my last semester of graduate work, upon the condition that he would allow me to start my new personal training business in his club. He thought about it for a minute and said, "Sure, I'll even be your first client".

Five months later, I came back, started my business at the same club that had fired me, and the rest is history. Instead of burning bridges, I turned it into the beginning of a new business from the very club that had just fired me five months earlier.

Client requests for my assistance demonstrated my expertise in my field as well as the level of customer satisfaction I was able to provide. Maintaining a positive relationship and effective communication with the owners under harsh conditions increased their belief in my credibility, reliability, and conscientiousness.

Instead of demonstrating anger, abusing the new management, or badmouthing them to others, I was able to reinforce the perception of my value as an asset to their new business.

Keep in mind that there are a lot more things that can come out of situations like these. If you have a bad attitude, criticize management, mention problems without attempting to find solutions, etc. your coworkers and employer will have plenty to say about you. If you are seen as someone who reduces the value of the business, team, or department, chances are that your reputation is going downhill fast.

Being seen as untrustworthy, rude, and critical will cause your professional contacts to discuss your behavior both inside and outside of work, resulting in the loss of potential work and advancement.

14

"YOU ARE THE ONLY ONE WHO TELLS ME WHAT TO DO...

...who I listen to." I remember the day my client told me this. I had just ordered up another round of grueling upper body exercises. He uttered these words through teeth clenched with determination and a stiff upper lip speckled with sweat.

This is a client who left no doubt as to his decision-making standards, his place in the world, and the value of his time. Because he listened to me, his health had improved immensely, as had the quality of his life.

Do your clients listen to you? We tend to listen to others to the degree that they listen to us. They tend to heed our words with the same weight and seriousness they feel we give to theirs.

Why do they need to listen to what you tell them to do? Their workout sessions with you are only a small part of their overall life, yet can have the largest impact...if and when they follow your other guidelines.

Have you talked to your clients about the importance of proper nutrition, stress reduction, and physical activity on their off-workout days? How they live their life when they are not working out with you has a direct bearing on the success they have as a result of working out with you.

Will they achieve their workout goals with you while they make poor lifestyle choices the remainder of the week? If they are static in their progress, how long will it be before they are no longer your client? If they don't heed the recommendations you make for the achievement of their goals, how will you be the hero you would have been if they followed your advice.

When you've really listened to their goals, their dreams, and their conversation about their life, you can see the bigger picture. When you are effective at helping them see that bigger picture and lay the cards out in front of them with a direction and a plan for success, they are more apt to listen and eagerly comply.

It's hard enough to get good clients and harder to retain them when they don't listen to you.

Do they have the desire to follow a healthy lifestyle?

Do they feel the information you are giving them has value to them, is it interesting to them?

Do they understand how it applies to their life and their workout outcomes?

Can they actually apply it to their lives or are there cross-purposes at work preventing effective compliance?

Do they have a spouse sabotaging their efforts, a demanding boss and long hours on the job, an eating disorder?

You need to know what you are up against to be able to tackle it.

To get their attention and make a strong impression with a client who doesn't listen, preface your statements by saying, "This is important to helping you achieve your goals. I need you to..." Tell them straight and crystal what it is they need to be doing, and why.

When you have listened, and understand them, you have a very good chance of having a client who lets you tell them what to do...and listens to you.

15

"A REAL LITTLE BUSINESS"

Perception is Reality. What is your clients' perception of your business? Whether you're running an outdoor boot camp or have an indoor facility, it's important to run your business in a professional manner.

When I started my business in the mid 80's, most trainers were "gym rats" without any formal education or business knowledge, just a bunch of "muscle heads" that liked to workout. One of the first things I did was to develop a formal business plan and formally incorporate Kansas City's original personal training center, and ran it like a real business. I hired an accountant and a lawyer; and I built a team of formally educated fitness professionals.

About three years into the business, as one of my clients was leaving, and several clients and trainers were mulling around the studio, she said to me "Wow, this is turning into a real little business, isn't it?" With that statement, it was clear that her perception of my business had been elevated to a higher level by the professional structure I had developed.

Sixty percent of small businesses – most of which fail – begin because the owners want to make money from a hobby. They see their recreational activities as social and financial opportunities and expect to enjoy spending the week engaged in their favorite activity. Businesses do not often succeed based on this idea because businesses have one purpose: to make money. To succeed financially, you do need to know your "hobby" inside and out – but that is a small part of running a business. Knowledge of accounting, marketing, customer service, and other business components are essential. If you are not able to handle these things yourself, you need to have the capital to hire accountants, attorneys, and great salespeople in order to run a real business.

Upon entering your establishment, an employee who can provide an established pricing structure based on detailed descriptions of everything that your business offers should greet potential clients. They should also be given brochures or printed packets detailing the information you give them. Included should be client recommendations, employee credentials and certifications, and your contact information. Most importantly, it should direct them to your website for additional information. If you don't have a website, your business is not taking advantage of a low-cost way to reach a large portion of potential customers.

The success or failure of your business is largely influenced by how it is perceived. These days, consumers are informed, knowledgeable about researching companies, and have expectations that you need to meet in order to even be considered as their choice provider.

Demonstrate knowledge, professionalism, training, and a past history of success and you will retain and increase your client base.

16

YOU KNOW THE PHYSICAL STUFF, BUT ARE YOU SMART TOO?

Is there more to you than meets the eye? I'd bet there is.

Are you sure your clients know?

Sometimes you have to let them know more about your business, because our clients tend to have tunnel vision. They see us as serving the main purpose for which we were hired. When they have been clients for any amount of time, they tend to forget all the wonderful programs and opportunities you offer, or perhaps you never told them.

We can become complacent and assume that everyone knows everything we know about what we provide. The reality is that we must educate and involve our clients about everything we offer and can do for them and their family and friends. If we don't, they will only know that you do what you do for them.

A personal training client who is also a CEO drove that point home to me one day. I had been giving him copies of my corporate wellness articles to read. One day, on my way to a meeting with his HR Director to discuss their Corporate Boot Camp I was setting up for them, our paths crossed in the lobby.

He introduced me to the business colleagues he was with and mentioned the articles I had written. His words hit home, "I knew you were good at the physical stuff, but I didn't know you were smart too."

What do your clients say about you or your club? Their perception of you is what they share with others. What they share with others is a testimonial to you as well as them. When they share information about you, the opportunity for a referral increases and a door opens to asking questions and seeking answers. Do you know what they are sharing about you?

Wiston Auden said, "Almost all of our relationships begin and most of them continue as forms of mutual exploitation, a mental or physical barter, to be terminated when one or both parties run out of goods."

Listen to your clients listen to you. If you only run your session and don't share other aspects of your business, your skills, the opportunities you have to help them in other ways, they won't know that you are smart too. Tell them, and show them too.

Assess your client relationships to see what they really know about you. Ask them to describe your club and its services. Listen to their responses.

Your relationship with your clients began with your need for an income and career combined with their need for guidance and instruction in physical fitness. A mutual benefit that served both of you well, as long as you delivered the goods.

As you grew your business, you introduced more 'goods' that you could deliver. Do all of your clients know this? Help them to be able to put it into words so they can be more effective spokespeople for you and your business.

Do this and you will be able to hear them say, "...and smart too!"

17

THEY WANT IT WHEN THEY ASK FOR IT

Has a client ever called you out? Mine did. It was years ago and my priorities changed in an instant.

I had always prided myself on knowing that I was focused on the client, their life, and their goals. Their needs were number one in my heart and my mind when we were in session.

That one day changed forever the way I do business. I had been training a valued long-time client. She is a delightful woman, energetic, intelligent, and very caring. A prominent member of society, influential people think highly of her. It was a rest period and she asked me for a towel.

I was bending over picking up a step. I acknowledged her desire for a towel while I was, in my opinion, clearing the area for the next moves, in the interest of her safety and space. Fifteen seconds it took, and then I went to get the towel.

As I handed her the towel, she shoved it back in my chest saying, "I wanted it when I asked for it!", and walked out.

Those words cut me to the quick with disbelief and confusion. I felt totally justified in taking 15 seconds to clear the gym floor before getting the towel. Fifteen seconds!

Remember Sir Isaac Newton's third law of physics the physics principle of propulsion…Every Action has an Equal and Opposite Reaction?

Where do you think my business would be today if I had become reactive instead of proactive? If I had tried to explain myself, dismiss her words, or dish it right back, would she have come back? Who would she have shared that with?

That day as I heard those stinging words from my valued client's lips, I instantly realized many things:

Different people have different focus, different definitions, different perceptions, and different priorities of the same event or circumstances. What I think to be the case, may not be what they think is the case. What I think of, as good business may not be what they think of as good business.

I chose to change the way I ran my fitness business and redefined how I focus on my clients. Actions do speak louder than words. My philosophy since that day is they want it when they want it. And I give it to them. That is what they pay me for, and that is what I will always deliver.

She called me later that day to apologize, calling it an "heiress moment". She was accustomed to getting things when she wanted them, the way she wanted them. I share this story with her permission and she is still my valued client with whom I have a wonderful working relationship.

Whether your client is actually a princess or not, each client deserves to be given what they want, when they ask for it. That's what they pay you for and that's how you retain clients.

18

"OLD IS OKAY AS LONG AS OLD IS CLEAN"

Have you ever marveled at the course your life or your business takes you? When you look back can you see those defining moments when you made a decision one way or the other, when you stood your ground, when you opted to take the risk or instead made a safer choice?

I woke up one morning recently marveling at the course my life and my business has taken me. A series of snapshot memories flooded my brain. I remembered watching Jack Lalanne's exercise show as a kid, thinking it was pretty cool. He was certainly a role model and inspiration as I entered the personal training world in 1986.

I related to him and his struggles early in my career. He went against the grain with a laser focus. He wasn't afraid to ruffle some feathers and to try new things. Much like Jack, I set my sites and plowed ahead.

Another image I saw was a few years back when a long time client walked in as I was on my hands and knees cleaning my favorite multi-station unit (which I have had repainted and recovered twice). We talked and I told him how special that unit was to me, even though it was from 1986. He nodded definitively and said, "Old is okay as long as old is clean." I've always remembered that comment.

What he was really saying was that he saw and appreciated the value I placed in my investment. Keeping my equipment clean, neat, and in good working order has served me well in my business. Saving money and preventing downtime as well as the reliability of good equipment helps me keep my businesses on track.

That client saw the value in the care I took with my equipment, and he also clearly saw the value that I placed in him and the training sessions I provided for him. His approval meant more to me than just a passing comment. Our clients talk to other people about important things in their life. What are your clients saying about you and the way you value and keep your business, equipment, and clients?

As I continued reflecting on "old" it occurred to me that our bodies need the same care as our equipment. I'm grateful that I have had the dedication to consistent and regular exercise throughout my life, no doubt influenced by Jack Lalanne, who, lived to be 96 years of age.

This day of reflection was my 49th birthday, still far from old. A wise man, Jack LaLanne, has been credited with saying, "People don't die of old age, they die of neglect." That same adage is true of business. Listen to your mentors, listen to your clients, listen to your own body, and then take action accordingly.

In another 24 years, I hope to show you my old multi-station still looking clean and new and working like a charm!

19

CONFESSIONS:
HOW I ACHIEVED SUCCESS IN SPITE OF MYSELF

I have spent my entire career doing everything 'wrong' according to the 'experts' and have still had great success in my businesses and my life. I agree whole-heartedly with those experts. In fact, in my fitness business-coaching program I encourage trainers to take those 'right' steps.

One key area where I have done it all 'wrong' is the area of working on my business, instead of in my business.

As I coach trainers with this advice, I still train clients myself, in addition to working on my businesses.

Am I being hypocritical?
Am I playing both sides of the fence afraid to step over?
Is it the money?
Why would I still be training clients?

Here's why. I have an incredibly supportive family. We work and play well together. I have built incredible relationships with clients I've had for 15, 18, 20 plus years. I have a social life with them. They have fed my business with referrals, income and support.

Our families have become a special part of each other's lives. They add something excellent and fruitful to my life and my business, regularly and deeply.

Some questions I've asked myself:

- Which clients do I choose to turn that 'special time' over to another trainer?
- Will I have to redefine my relationships with them if I am not training them?
- Am I ready to let go of the reins and listen to my own advice?
- Do I really "need" to?

My life and my businesses are about relationships first. That was my plan and how I grew my business. I've built incredibly satisfying relationships and they have helped me to succeed. People believed in me and the services I offered. My relationships with people are the reason for my success. Without them, I would just be another great trainer that no one has heard of.

Some things you must consider if you want to 'do it all wrong' and succeed in spite of yourself:

- Know yourself and your limitations. It is hard enough to bounce back from burnout, and even more so from repeated bouts of burnout. You must be able to say STOP and get away to rejuvenate yourself before you get to that point of burnout.

- Know which relationships help nurture and support your dreams, and willingly pick up some of your slack (and you will be leaving slack if you do things the 'wrong' way). Nurture and embrace those relationships. They will make all the difference in your success.

- Know your direction, ultimate goals, stepping stone goals, and time frames. Create a plan for it all.

- Live within your means and plan your days.

- Work your plan faithfully until your goals change.

The earlier in your fitness business you start working ON it, in addition to IN it, the better your chance of developing and choosing the types of relationships that will help you build a strong and steady business and carry you into your future.

20

LEAVE A LEGACY –
A TRIBUTE TO JACK LALANNE

Does a person who leaves a legacy of change, social and individual improvement, and self-challenge have to be larger than life? Maybe, but they don't start out that way. The person who leaves a legacy could be you, me, or the trainer down the street.

Each of us has the opportunity to leave a legacy that makes all the difference in the life of at least one individual.

Jack LaLanne was larger than life and was called "The Godfather of Fitness".   As a youngster his muscles, his abilities, and his fortitude mesmerized me. Our TV set allowed me to workout with him and to feel his encouragement like he was right there with me. He inspired me, along with millions of others. I picked up his gauntlet of challenge and pursued fitness as my daily way of life, fitness as my business, and fitness as my mission.

It was Jack's inspiration, his lead, and his action that led to the development of health clubs and fitness centers as we know them today. Jack's focused pursuit of purpose and his undying belief in the power of a strong body helped propel exercise science and natural health forward.

The power we have to change people's lives is very real and much more than simply training people to exercise.

That power is held in a smile, a nod, a gentle push, a kick in the butt, a pat on the back, a simple "Let me show you." and a shared 'well done!' That is the power to propel and that power is held by each and every one of us.

Jack grew into his legacy by doing and giving, and doing some more. He first had to find his passion and purpose and then he pursued them relentlessly, increasing his knowledge with a combination of schooling and practical action on himself. With every new success, he would strive for more.

He saw the lack of means and method, so he designed equipment to help people achieve their specific fitness goals. His weight selectors and cables are still in use. His ideas evolved into bands and tubes - more lightweight, affordable, and easy to use by the average person. Providing a means to achieve success, offering the encouragement to pursue that success, living that success by example, all with purpose and love…isn't that what a legacy is about?

At the end of our lives, when we can turn around and see the ripple effect of our actions on the lives of others, will we be surprised? The countless people whose perspectives we shifted into hope by spending that little bit of extra time showing them how to achieve something we thought was so simple…the countless people whose hope escalated when we worked with them, side by side, to help them see, feel, and taste success…the countless people whose successes we recognized and applauded, feeding their passion and determination for more…and the legacies those individuals are creating because we pursued our passion and gave of ourselves…will you be surprised?

There is always one more challenge awaiting us, one more person we can inspire, one more thing we can do...Jack LaLanne taught us much more than how to grow a strong and healthy body. He taught us to share and to care, to never say 'never', and to reach outside our perceived limitations because we CAN.

Thank you, Jack, for leaving a legacy of possibility, inspiration, and achievement while being an example that we may follow in building and leaving our own legacies.

21

USE YOUR MARKETING TO EDUCATE

"The aim of marketing is to know and understand the customer so well the product or service fits him and sells itself."

— Peter F. Drucker

As we all know, marketing can help you get new clients. Did you know that marketing can help you build a better relationship with the clients you already have? And that it can make them more committed to sticking with you and your training program?

Education-Based Marketing is the right type of marketing to help you achieve significant results. This type of marketing is based on educating your customers about the best way to choose the products and services that meet their needs. Every client has something to learn about your business – such as how training works with nutrition, basic anatomy and physiology, how to tell if your trainer is getting the results you want, etc.

When you educate your clients, you are adding value to your services. Also, because you're teaching them objectively, you will quickly build a strong foundation of trust since providing information isn't a sales pitch. They will see you as both a trainer and a reliable source of information, and this will keep them coming back. Educating your clients will make them loyal, satisfied, and more compliant. By the questions they ask as you teach them about the process and a few subtle questions of your own, you can quickly determine the customers' needs and find the right services and products to deliver exactly what they're looking for.

The key to success with this type of marketing is that you provide up-to-date, relevant, and accurate information. You need to be seen as an expert in your field; and your clients need to feel sure that they can come to you with questions and get better answers than they can find on the internet. So, you need to create a plan for accomplishing these goals, as you would with any other type of marketing strategy.

"A clear vision, backed by definite plans, gives you a tremendous feeling of confidence and personal power."
– Brian Tracy

Begin by asking yourself questions about how you can achieve credibility, accurate information aggregation, and position yourself as an expert. You need to think about the types of clients you have, what kind of information is most helpful to them and what they are most likely to ask, and then you need to create a detailed plan for accumulating this information and easily acquiring the results of new studies and breakthroughs in training.

It helps to use reliable sources, both within your industry and outside it, so that your clients can verify your information if they wish. Providing your clients with complex and intricate information will exponentially increase your credibility and the extra value that your clients believe they are getting.

Choose your own reliable sources of information, create a plan to stay updated (Such as RSS feeds), and remember that data and statistics pack a serious punch.

Make sure you don't forget your ultimate goal – which is to deliver exactly what your clients want…and a little more.

22

DO WE HAVE A DEAL?

I believe in adding on value rather than cutting my price.

Like you, I offer a fair price for my services and give clients every penny's worth.

Communicating that value to a prospect is easy when they are almost ready to sign. Adding on an unexpected, unpublicized product or service related to the one they are looking at purchasing can clinch the deal and create the goodwill that will help produce a really good client.

How do you communicate that value to a prospect who is sitting on the fence and telling you that price is the only reason they haven't signed the deal yet? Obviously price is not the only factor, or they would be gone. There is something else they haven't said.

Many prospects that don't sign are weighing pros and cons. Do you know what those pros and cons are? If not, ask them. They have already determined they NEED this program, or at least something like it. They know the cost/benefit ratio. They DESIRE the results this program of yours will give them.

Yet they still sit on the fence. What is their unspoken obstacle? They KNOW you will deliver what you say you will deliver; after all, you have been running a successful business and they see the activity and the testimonials. Deep in the recesses of their mind and their heart, they know they will not commit. They know they will probably not follow through. At the very least, they have doubts about their performance, not yours.

Explore their pros and cons with them. Most people will not readily or easily admit to their lack of true commitment. They will acknowledge, however, their busy schedules, multiple commitments, and possible interferences with their attendance in your program. They will acknowledge tight finances, and many other factors surrounding the main issue they are not speaking.

Have them picture their life after participation in your program. Help them speak it real. Then ask what they need to get there. Their answers may surprise you. Or they may be clueless.

If they are looking for weight loss you can share studies show the people who kept daily food diaries lost twice the weight or more compared with those who did not keep records. If they lean forward or their eyes widen, you know you have hit close to home.

You have given them tangible information on a course of success they know they can do. They know they can write down their food, whereas they are not sure they will go to your gym or studio as scheduled. They may realize that this is the one thing that will help them over the hump and into the groove.

A pedometer is another great added value. The bottom line is that it's not just a product or service you are providing, but a means of achieving sustainable accountability.

Don't sell yourself short. Add something of value that will help them feel more capable in their quest for success.

Do we have a deal?

23

ACCENTUATE THE POSITIVE

" If you think you can do a thing or think you can't do a thing, you're right.

— Henry Ford

Henry Ford was right on the money. While you can't control everything that happens to you, you do have 100% control over how you respond. By recognizing how limiting beliefs hold you back, you safeguard yourself from falling victim to these in the future.

Researchers have discovered many amazing things about the relationship between the mind and body that impact health and healing. We know that each person has a unique mind/body relationship. As with all relationships, you can experience synchronicity and disagreements.

There is one fundamental secret to success in achieving breakthroughs: Your brain won't make you a liar. What you believe is created by your own thoughts. Your thoughts and beliefs will align your speech, actions, and body to produce the results you expect. Here is this concept in action:

During one of my regular workouts with my son David, I asked him how many times he could flip a 6 foot, 400 lb. tractor tire. He thought about it and said, "Four". David, a strong, capable athlete, then flipped the tire four times and was both physically and emotionally spent.

The next time, David felt that he didn't know how many times he could flip the tire, and decided to find out. When he lifted the restrictions he placed on himself, he was unstoppable. David expanded his thinking and allowed his mind/body relationship to grow with the simple words, "Let's see what I can do!"

Clients with self-sabotaging beliefs don't always realize how often they are reinforcing those beliefs. When your conscious mind retrieves information from your subconscious, it will pull the information you tell it to, just like a search engine. So, when clients think they can't do something and you ask them why they can't, their minds will pull supporting information that may not be realistic, practical, or useful. The most familiar limiting beliefs are:

I can't do it
My family is overweight
No matter what I do, I can't lose weight

These limiting beliefs serve no useful purpose because they only serve to prevent clients from achieving their goals.

Counteracting these negative thoughts requires careful construction. Negative reinforcement doesn't work because the mind fights too hard against it. Push clients to pay close attention to every improvement they make. Then, develop statements based on how they feel after they work out, or when they are able to increase their max weight or cardio limit. So, to reaffirm their commitments, replace those nasty negative thoughts with reminders of their improvements and how great it feels to achieve these milestones. Also, continually emphasize that they are getting stronger every day and are actively pursuing their goals.

Successful clients prove your effectiveness as a trainer. Not to mention, they complain less and are more fun to work with. Find positive ways to encourage your clients and help them overcome these obstacles, and you will see them achieve more than they thought possible.

24

ARE YOU A SEXY-MAKER
OR HEALTH PRODUCER?

As Personal Trainers, we see what is happening with the decline in the health of Americans today and we have the tools to turn that tide instantly, moving America back to health and wellness. Why aren't most trainers actively pursuing the health and wellness message?

There are generally two schools of thought about exercise. One group loves it and thrives on it; the other group eyes it with distaste, ignorance, or lack of interest (this group is much larger).

Our profession has increased in popularity over the years with this first group. The focus has been on the exterior of the body (from "their" perspective), "cool" and scant apparel, excitement and sweat. The end result is to create a new body shape, a sexier body, or a muscular body. The inferred message is that you will be more popular, happier, more attractive to the opposite sex, or a better athlete.

This image does nothing for the percentage of our population in the other group, so we have effectively cut off communications with the second group who do not see the need for a sexy body in their life.

The truth is that they DO need regular exercise in their life, but not for the reasons we have advertised and marketed. They need regular exercise for their health and quality of life because regular exercise is what their body needs to give them that health and quality of life.

Can a profession suddenly change the direction of its message and purpose mid-stream, while maintaining its current message? Not possible. As complex as the human brain is, it likes simplicity and black and white.

When the doctor tells a patient to get regular exercise and proper nutrition, and the patient perceives the doctor as a "fixer of problems by dispensing magic pills", the patient would rather just have a pill.

Some in the medical profession have aligned themselves with an image that has removed self-care accountability from the average person and laid that accountability at the feet of the doctor to get them well and keep them healthy.

When you look at how the majority of our population views the roles of doctors and personal trainers, you start to understand that the depth of our health crisis in America runs much deeper than mere statistics. Misunderstanding is woven into the very core of our culture.

How do we transform our image from sexy-maker to health-producer so we can capture that market and make a real difference in the health of our citizens?

We must position ourselves as having a separate program that is marketed strictly to health benefits and make it available at a time and place where people are thinking about and need to do something about their health. That position is ideally in the workplace.

On-site Corporate Fitness is more than simply a niche market. It is the means and the method of educating the American public to the value of Personal Trainers and professionally written exercise programs in helping them regain their health and wellness.

25

A CORPORATE BOOT CAMP IN EVERY BUSINESS

Every business, large or small, can and should have a corporate boot camp active within its walls, or at the very least, a stone's throw away. The workplace is a logical location and time for a boot camp. The job, career, or work life is fully one third of the average American's life. Another third is spent sleeping, and the remaining third is the time they use to get everything else done that they want and need to do.

We live in a world that moves very fast. Micro this, instant that. The pace is hectic, the demands are great, and stress is high. Business needs employees to be fully present, alert, and productive. Those qualities can be truly difficult to achieve when a person is unhealthy, chronically ill, or absent.

Business has a vested interest in maintaining employee health. You have the ability, skills, and knowledge to provide it.

The average participation level at workplace boot camps runs between 25% and 45%. The ideal number of participants for a trainer is 10 - 20 per session. Our ideal starting point is with businesses that have 100 or more employees because of these facts.

If a smaller business has just 10 employees who are already committed to wellness or fitness, go for it. You won't have to worry about fall off and you'll probably see a lot more energy.

Whether the business has 10 employees, 50, or 100, trainers need to maintain their professionalism and their corporate processes.

On-site programs are most effective. It's been shown to be less likely for employees to venture out elsewhere to exercise, and most feel short of time as it is. You can use a conference room, warehouse, parking lot, yard area, or anywhere else that may be appropriate and available.

Start with a **Needs Assessment Survey**. You and the business will both have a picture to work from.

Use body weight and/or limited equipment. It's easy and fast to pick up afterward.

Plan on a half-hour class, with 15 minutes before and after for motivating and answering questions.

Be aware of sound levels. Music, pounding and noise can be disruptive while others are working or holding a phone conference nearby.

Trainer does the record keeping and reports to management. Assessment every 12 weeks is a good idea.

A simple guideline for pricing your corporate boot camp starts with your base hourly rate. Ours is $200. When we run a half-hour program the value is $100. If there are 10 people in the program session that means $10 per person x 12 weeks totals $120 per person for a 12 week corporate boot camp session.

Our all-inclusive pricing also covers the nutrition component of meal planning and grocery lists. If you job out other services that you don't handle yourself, you can choose to let that company do the quoting and billing.

Newbie Trainers Checklist - Here are some must know basics when first starting a corporate boot camp program or you may find yourself working for next to nothing.

- Know your customer. Are they sedentary? Do they spend their days pushing and no pulling? You will get a heath history on each, yet there will be trends in the job functions at different businesses. Know these so you can plan your exercise workouts accordingly.

- Be clear about what is and isn't included in your price and what your payment schedule is. Be clear about what your responsibilities are, as well as what you expect from management and employees.

- It's all about them. Make sure their needs, concerns, and desires are addressed. You are working for them. Do your job and do it well. Leave your personal life at home. Focus on the client while on-site.

- Scout the building out with the owner or manager signing the check. Make sure you both agree on a location(s) and time(s) for the corporate boot camp workouts. Nothing leaves a bitter taste than a miscommunication in business.

- Get it in writing. A completed contract includes dates, times, locations, session start and end dates, costs, payment schedule, session expectations, and session length.

- Remember who your client is. You are accountable to the company. They are paying the bill.

- Always respect individual privacy rights, even though the client is the company.

- Plan your 12 sessions in advance. Plan your email topics in advance. Have your website up and running in advance.

- Do not add to the paperwork load for HR. You do most of the paperwork.

- Be where you said you would be when you said you would.

- Enjoy yourself and have fun!

We offer a complete checklist to trainers free for the asking at info@aycfit.com.

The majority of corporate boot camps are run during the lunch hour if they have shower facilities. Employees will workout for a half hour and then they have the other half hour to change and eat, then they are back at their desk or workstation. If there are no showers available, they will do their workouts after work. This is a major discussion point that must be covered early on in the sales process.

The business owner wants to know that it is not costing him to offer this program. He or she must know that it is not disrupting the workplace or the work schedule. When the program starts, the employees must know this also. One bad apple can spoil the whole bunch.

Make sure you run a tight ship and follow the guidelines that you establish with the business owner. If you are running back to back programs with the same company, make sure you are moving them in and out exactly on schedule. One slip up by you and the employee gets off track with the boss.

The confidence and respect the business owner has for you is in direct proportion to how well you cover your bases up front, run your program, follow the guidelines you both agreed upon, as well as the results you get. The ease with which they renew their contract with you is also in direct proportion to those same factors.

It is a big deal for a business owner to hold a boot camp for its employees. It is an honor for you to be considered as their trainer. When you respect that honor and do a very good job for them, they will not hesitate to refer and recommend you to their network of business owner acquaintances.

With those referrals, your program and processes will carry you far and wide into the incredible world of corporate boot camps.

26

THE CORPORATE BOOT CAMP CRAZE

In 1986 I began my career as a corporate and community wellness supervisor in Kansas City. That was also the same year I began my personal fitness training business. I was fortunate to have had the opportunity to work with more than 64 of Kansas City's most progressive thinking corporations. I call them progressive because, way back in 1986, these companies were already committed to creating a wellness environment for their employees.

We provided these companies with programs that included healthy eating, stress management, smoking cessation, aerobics classes and, my favorite, the Kansas City Corporate Challenge. Corporate Challenge was an annual event that allowed companies to compete against each other in more than 30 different athletic events such as basketball, bowling, track and field, and triathlon. Today there are more than 100 companies that participate in KCCC.

Fast-forward more than 25 years and instead of aerobics classes, you have corporate boot camps. I see a lot of similarities with the aerobics craze of the early and mid 80's and the boot camp craze of today. The high intensity workouts we did back then incorporated a lot of the same movements that are used in today's boot camp workouts. We didn't use sandbags and kettle bells back then, but there were a lot of burpees and plyometrics.

Another big difference between the 1980's and today...no more spandex!

With the recent influx of personal trainers entering the corporate fitness market, I've been getting a lot of calls and emails asking how to get started. As Chet Holmes explains in, his "Ultimate Sales" book, there are seven steps to every sale.

1. Establish Rapport
2. Qualify the Buyer (Find the Need)
3. Build Value
4. Create Desire
5. Overcome Objections
6. Close the Sale
7. Follow Up

There's really no difference between selling personal training and corporate boot camps. The hardest part is getting the attention of the client.

How do you get their attention in the first place?

It's all about marketing. You've got to be where your potential client lives his or her life. Whether it's in the publications they're reading, the TV show's they're watching or the restaurants they're eating, you've got to have a presence.

Once you have their attention, you've begun the process of Establishing Rapport. Recently, while doing some market research, one of my long time clients said to me "If I didn't know you, you'd never have gotten the chance to present your corporate boot camp program to my company." Harsh words? No, just the reality of today's fast paced "get it done" yesterday lifestyle. The truth of the matter is that it was the ultimate compliment. I have worked with his family for more than 20 years and have developed an incredible friendship and business relationship that benefits both parties.

Because of the relationship I have developed with him and his family, I was able to secure a corporate contract that has allowed me to expand my business to different parts of the country.

The key is that *I already had his attention* when I approached his company about my corporate boot camp program. Remember step one of the seven steps of sales, Establish Rapport. All of my clients are my friends, and each of them is a potential source of added business from referrals in my personal training and corporate boot camp businesses.

If you are a personal trainer trying to break into the corporate fitness market, you've already got a great head start...
...your current client base.

Use what no one else, except you – your list.

Leverage each and every one of your clients.

All of your clients or their spouses work, right?

You've got a good relationship with them, don't you?

The social proof is already there. Your program works, why not share it with others?

The research is overwhelming when it comes to workplace wellness programs lowering health care costs for businesses so, steps two, three, and four of the sales process should fall right into place.

Step number five can be a little trickier. How do you overcome objections? Let me give you one example.

When I first proposed our boot camp program to a corporate client, I was told that too many of their employees traveled and wouldn't benefit from our workouts. Since my personal training business had an online component, I suggested that we add it to the company's program. That way, they could take their workouts and meal plan anywhere they traveled. Problem solved, objection overcome, contract signed.

Perhaps the second most important step in the sales process is number seven, the Follow Up. That's right, it's not finished **after** you close the sale.

Did you know that it costs six times more to get a new client than to keep and/or sell something additional to a current client? If the hardest thing we do is to get the attention of a new client, doesn't it make sense to make a special effort to keep your current clients happy?

There are several things you can do, as part of your follow up, such as sending a monthly newsletter or greeting cards, holding client appreciation events or giving them small gifts that are relevant to your business. These are very important tactics but, more importantly, there has to be an open line of communication. The decision makers have to be comfortable enough with you to tell you when something's wrong.

Apathy is your worst enemy.

The best-case scenario would be to have the decision makers participating in your corporate boot camps. That way they can see exactly what's going on with your program. There's an energy that's hard to explain with these corporate boot camps. The participants in these programs bond with each other. It's almost like a fraternity. If the decision maker doesn't participate, you must make a special effort to keep the lines of communications open. I always tell the participants to share their experience with the management of the corporation.

Nothing sells your product like enthusiastic campers.

Recently, one of my boot camp instructors told me that one of his campers came to him after the class and said "Next week I'm on vacation, but I'm coming in so I don't have to miss my workouts." Now **that's** the kind of advocate you want spreading the word about your business.

27

WHAT MAKES A GREAT PERSONAL FITNESS TRAINER?

Whenever I read a book or article, the first thing I do is ask, "Why is this person qualified to write this?"

Before reading, I always look at the bio at the end to see if I want to continue reading. If you do that same thing, I'm going to answer this chapter title question right now.

It's about building relationships.

I opened Kansas City's original personal fitness training center in 1986 and, as of 2011, have personally trained over 45,000 one-hour private sessions during the past 26 years.

It's about building relationships.

I stopped taking new clients in 1994 so I could focus on my core 20 clients, yet my business continued to grow. Why? Simply because I have an incredible staff that schedules new clients regularly.

It's about building relationships.

My mission was, and still is, about building relationships with clients who are committed to a healthy lifestyle, including regular exercise. I have 17 clients that have had the same weekly time slots with me for over 23 years - and another three that have for over 18 years. Building relationships translates to client retention and a growing, successful business.

Have you ever wondered what makes a great personal fitness trainer? What separates a mediocre personal trainer from an incredible personal trainer? Important questions, right?

Here are the four "P's" that I believe make for a great personal trainer.

1. PASSION
2. PERSUASION
3. PERSEVERENCE
4. PATIENCE

PASSION...do you have it? An enthusiastic trainer is motivational and clients respond to that. If you don't have passion for this industry, you might as well save yourself the time and stop reading now, because that's where it all begins.

I believe it's the single most important component to being a great trainer. It's more important than the alphabet soup after your name (your formal education and certifications), more important than the years of experience you've accumulated and certainly more important than being able to lift 300 lbs. or having six-pack abs.

Now, don't misunderstand me, I'm not saying that education and experience aren't important, I have a master's degree myself, and you should be a walking role model for your clients. What I'm saying is that those are secondary to the infectious power of passion.

Passion is any powerful or compelling emotion or feeling, and it can manifest itself in many different ways. Here's where you get a bonus "P"…Personality. It is about building relationships and connecting emotionally with your client. Understanding, compassion and confidentiality…no one respects a blabbermouth. Clients need to be able to trust you.

I'm the "high energy" kind of trainer, and sure, that comes from a lot of passion, but some of the best trainers I've known have a more subtle kind of passion to which their clients respond. There's no right or wrong way when it comes to passion, it's just critical that you walk it, talk it, and live it.

You can't fake passion, and you can't learn it either. You either have it or you don't.

- Do you wake up in the morning looking forward to going to work?
- Do you greet every client with a smile and a positive comment?
- After each appointment, do you send your client away with a comment of affirmation?

If not, you need to rethink your strategy.

Now, I'm not going to lie, and tell you that I've woken up every morning during the past 9,490 days with 100% zeal or fervor. But, I can honestly say that at least 8,541 of those mornings I have. If you're doing the math, that's 90%. I use the 90% rule with my clients and tell them that if you follow your plan at least 90% of the time, you'll see amazing results. Even when you're not at 100%, your innate passion for what you do will kick in and your clients will never know the difference.

PERSUASION – Do your clients listen to you? Are you convincing?

The analogy I like to use is a teacher in a classroom. The trainer is a teacher. You must be persuasive to get your message across. You're going to hear every excuse in the book as to why your client can't or won't do something you ask. This is where your formal education and the powers of persuasion will come in handy, because you must make a good argument to counter their excuses.

The act of persuading is the act of influencing the mind by arguments or reasons offered.

If a client tells you they don't have time for a workout, you should have a scripted comeback ready to deliver. You must have conviction while making your argument. You've got to believe what you're telling them is true. And, you must present a factual and compelling case.

Part of persuasion is your presentation. You can't be caught off guard. If you've been training for any length of time, you've heard all the excuses. Be prepared. Be ready to strike back with confidence, reason and facts.

Finally, if you can't persuade a client to be motivated, say, "You're fired." Don't let frustration overtake you or your client. When you have a genuine passion for training and the ability to persuade, you have to give it your all. You are the teacher...it is your responsibility to motivate.

Be mindful that not every trainer is right for every client. It must be a win/win situation.

PERSEVERANCE – A steady persistence in a course of action or purpose in spite of difficulties, obstacles, or discouragement.

We've all had clients that have gone through tough times, or have been discouraged by one thing or another. Maybe your client only lost one pound over the course of a week, and thought they should have lost three. Or perhaps they're going through personal problems in their lives, and feel the need to share those issues with you.

Are you a good listener? If not, you need to remember that you have two ears and only one mouth so learn to listen twice as much as you talk.

When a client gets discouraged, or gets off track because of personal reasons, it's easy to give up on them and go looking for new clients. Are you a quitter? Or, do you confront issues head on and preserver? We're in this business to help people. Remember, it's all about building relationships. It is not about you.

Constancy, dedication, determination and endurance are all synonyms for perseverance.

Are you dedicated to your clients?

Are you determined, and do you have the endurance to see them through tough times? If so, you shouldn't have any difficulty with the last "P" – Patience.

PATIENCE – We've all heard the saying that "patience is a virtue". As a personal trainer it is a good and admirable quality to have. It really goes hand in hand with perseverance. If you think about it, patience really implies qualities of calmness, stability and persistent courage in trying circumstances.

Have you ever had a client that just couldn't "get it" when you tried to explain how to do something? We've all been there, and it can be frustrating. Just because it comes natural to you doesn't mean it's easy for your clients.

A true measure of patience is when you can suppress restlessness or annoyance when you are confronted with a slow learner. Never show your frustration with them. Always remain calm and relaxed when explaining something to them for the 4th, 5th, even 10th time. Remember, the client has paid for your time and undivided attention. A slow learner who may not possess the perfect athletic skills will get even more satisfaction when they "get it." Your patience will pay big dividends.

Are you building relationships?

Ask yourself the following four questions, and be honest when you answer.

1. Are you passionate about what you do?
2. Do you have the power of persuasion?
3. How persistent are you when it comes to what you desire?
4. Are you patient with your clients?

The first "P" PASSION is innate, but I believe the other three "P's" can be developed. Some trainers will have an easier time than others, but they can be developed.

Start building relationships today!

28

EDUCATION MATTERS

Hire personality and passion first, and then teach them to be good trainers, right? Sorry, but in my opinion that's just wrong. I know it's almost sacrilegious to say, because some of the top trainers in our industry preach that mantra, but I stand by my statement.

Hire education first, then personality and passion.

Every time this subject comes up I end up ruffling some feathers. It isn't my intention; it's just my opinion. I didn't even hire myself until I completed my master's degree.

Don't get me wrong, I'm not saying you should only hire trainers with their master's degree in exercise science, but they should be well trained and qualified before you allow them to work with clients. At the very least a top tier group like ACSM, ACE, AFAA, NASM, or NCSA should certify them.

Nearly two-thirds of the 2,700 certified trainers interviewed in a National Board of Fitness Examiners survey admitted knowing trainers they considered incompetent.

A study of health-and-fitness professionals published in the Journal of Strength and Conditioning Research found that trainers who had five years of experience but no college degree scored an average of 44 % on a test of basic fitness knowledge. Those with at least a bachelor's degree in exercise science scored an average of 68 %. Trainers with an ACSM or NSCA certification got 85 percent, while those with other certifications or none at all came in at 36 percent.

Education matters. As an industry we can do better. Our goal should be to raise the professional and ethical standard of our industry, not lower it. My concern is that we're too busy trying to entertain our clients rather than provide them with the proper guidance they really need.

Deana Melton, assistant professor at North Carolina Agricultural & Technical State University, has been interviewing club managers for an upcoming study on trainer qualifications. Some of the responses included; "We know it's important to hire quality trainers, but we... have to pay them more, and that cuts into our profit too much." (According to the U.S. Bureau of Labor Statistics, the average personal trainer makes $25,190 per year. The average hourly wage for a trainer at a chain club is $24.42.) She also found that some clubs hire college students—and not necessarily those with exercise-related majors—as trainers in exchange for free membership.

Your clients are the most valuable assets you have. Why would you risk putting them in the hands of someone without the proper qualifications because they have a good personality, or just to save a few bucks?

When I began AYC back in 1986, personal training, as an industry, included a lot of "gym rats" just trying to make an extra buck at the club. I believed then, and still do today, that raising the bar, as it relates to the "science" of personal training, was important. The art of personal training is important too, and that's where personality and passion come in.

If you want longevity in this industry, you must bring the science and art together.

29

AN OBSERVATION IN IRONY

Boot camp-style workouts are very trendy these days, and technology-based fitness continues to gain in popularity too.

Kind of interesting that two of the hottest trends in our industry couldn't be more diametrically opposed, isn't it? 'Old-School' Boot Camp Workouts and Technology-based fitness are both gaining in popularity, with no end in sight.

It's the movie Rocky IV all over again. That's right; Rocky Balboa versus Ivan Drago, old school verses state-of-the-art.

I won't lie, I loved the Rocky movies. I was a sixteen year-old high-school wrestler when the first Rocky movie made its 1976 debut.

Early morning workouts, drinking raw eggs and rooting for the underdog became a way of life for many young athletes, including me. By the way, skip the raw eggs...they're better and safer scrambled.

There are many memorable moments from the Rocky series, but the most relevant to this article is from the fourth installation, when Rocky goes to the Soviet Union to avenge the death of Apollo Creed at the hands of Ivan Drago.

Rocky trains for the fight by carrying logs, chopping wood and pulling a sleigh through the snow. Sounds familiar if you've participated in a boot camp workout class, doesn't it?

Drago, on the other hand, is attached to electrodes and is constantly monitored by computers, and works out with ultra hi-tech equipment.

Quite a contrast, isn't it?

So, the question is...which way is better, old school boot camp workouts or techno-fitness?

Would you rather be outside, flipping tires, pushing sleds, tossing medicine balls and swinging kettle bells or inside, going from machine to machine, like a robot, with a key card and heart monitor?

Well, I don't mind wearing a heart monitor every now and then, but I'd much rather be outside breathing fresh air. You can have the technology; my vote is for the boot camps!

30

FIND YOUR 4:00 A.M.

I've said it before and I'll say it again, 4:00 a.m. is my friend. I'm reminded of that every morning I walk outside to get the newspaper and look around to a world of no distractions, no hustle and bustle, and no interruptions. I know there are a lot of trainers that cringe when I say that, and the point of this is not about getting up early, it's about finding YOUR OWN 4:00 A.M.

You see that's the time of day when I'm at my peak as far as productivity goes. It's when I write most of my articles, do strategic planning, and get things done. And, that's what it's all about, isn't it, getting things done?

When are you at your peak?

What time of day do you do your best work?

When can you GET THINGS DONE?

Figure out what works best for you and block out those times to work on your business.

I also block off Tuesday and Thursday afternoons. That is the best time for me to catch up on meetings, phone calls, emails, blogs, and anything to do with people, because they are up and about. Those afternoons are time I can wrap up projects, begin new projects, find answers, discover new things, meet new people, and work on what I need to work on.

We have all been given 24 hours each day. We all have the power to choose how we use those hours. I have taken my hopes and dreams, and set them to paper as goals with a plan of action and a timeline. I have found the time, and made the time to pursue and achieve them. I hold myself accountable first to myself, and then to all the people who will be positively affected by those completed goals.

My 4:00 a.m. helps me be proactive, manage my time, get more accomplished, and spend more time with my family and friends. It helps me reduce stress. By the time the rest of the world is awake and just getting moving, I have things checked off my list for the day. I have a renewed sense of purpose. I have more time available later to go have lunch with my family, or to fit in something that may unexpectedly occur that I want to deal with. I have a clear brain to focus on my training sessions, on my meetings, and all my activities throughout the day.

The most important thing my 4:00 a.m. gives me is the ability to work ON my business, not IN my business.

I wouldn't trade my 4:00 a.m. for anything. That time I spend has been an investment in my business, my future, and me. It has been the door to many windows of opportunity, the key to my productivity, and the foundation of my entrepreneurial lifestyle. The consistency of my 4:00 a.m. uninterrupted time, my Tuesday and Thursday afternoons, and my nightly planning of the next day's activities, all help keep me on track without losing time, without hesitating, without doubt.

When is your 4:00 a.m.? The time when you are thinking clearly and quickly?

The time when you can have an hour of uninterrupted time to yourself to accomplish some of the important tasks on your list, in your goals, your plans?

The best investment you can make in yourself is to allow yourself that time.

Find it. Make it.

Your larger, bolder future is depending on it.

31 SIMPLE WAYS TO OVER-DELIVER

Over-delivering is business as usual in my book.

It is second nature to me to give clients more than they expect. I'm telling you now; it's a lot easier than it sounds. It may seem like some mysterious, expensive proposition that will cut into your time, your resources, and your bottom line. Don't worry, it doesn't. It only enhances all that and more.

It is surprisingly simple to over deliver to your personal training clients. One word of warning. Each and every method and means of over delivering must include some type of relationship. If it is done without relationship, it has little value. If it has little value, there is no "over deliver". I'll show you what I mean.

Let me share a mere 32 ways with you...there are hundreds...Here are some of the ways I over deliver...Remember...it's the little things that count.

Little Things
  1. Smile. Who wants to deal with a sourpuss?
  2. Say their name when speaking to them. That's a big one. Use it as you would with your best friend.
  3. Bring them their water. Refill their glass before they want it.

4. Introduce them to others warmly and enthusiastically.

Big Things

5. Use their testimonial on your website (with their permission).
6. Mention their achievements in your next local media interview (with their permission).
7. Tell them specifically what they have achieved and let them know that you are proud of them. Let them know that YOU know how much effort they put in to their achievement.
8. Explain how you can help their kids gain confidence against bullying with your exercise program.

Tangible Things

9. T-shirt, or other apparel. Something they can be proud to wear, that makes them one of "us" at this gym.
10. Pedometer. Something useful and functional that will help directly with their program and their wellness lifestyle.
11. Do a cross promotion with a local shoe or athletic store and give them a huge discount coupon from that store.

Intangible Things

12. Listen. They want you to hear them. They want to know that you know them.
13. Care. If they are in the midst of turmoil, let them know that you care. If a spouse dies, send a card and go to the funeral.
14. Relate to them. Be a real person, not a machine.

15. Wink at them. Acknowledge the extra effort your client puts in.

Educational/Informative Things
16. Print client handouts in areas they are interested in.
17. Talk with their doctor. If they are special populations, let them know when they are on track w/doctors knowledge.
18. Research and study. Share with them the latest findings in whatever area you are working with them on.
19. Share with them a new recipe or flavor combination (i.e.: honey and cinnamon on toast)

Time Things
20. Show them something special - specific exercises or stretches geared toward low back pain, easier sleep, etc.
21. Offer to go to their kid's school for show and tell or to speak and demo.
22. Offer to do a lunch and learn for their church or social group - you just may get some new clients in the process.
23. Ask them specifically if there is anything you can do for them.

Caring/Sharing Things
24. Remember their birthday, or their anniversary of working with you.
25. Give them a flower for Mother's Day (during that week) or Bosses Day (explaining that you work for them)

26. Give them a brochure or newspaper article to a place in their field of interest that they may not be aware of.
27. Celebrate with them - write a congratulations note on a banana (clean yellow skin, use a pen lightly) and present it to them.

Above and Beyond the Call of Duty Things
28. Surprise them with a chair massage.
29. Create a poster or sign that recognizes personal bests and achievements.
30. Have their name embroidered on one of your shirts or sweatshirts
31. Celebrate when they achieve the dress or pant size they wanted to get to. Cross promote with a popular clothing store and give them a discount coupon.

Some factors you need to know.

Your time, your knowledge, your skills, your words, your answers, all have value to a client - if you are a professional.

They know how much they are paying, they assume they know how you treat a regular client, and they know how you treat them. You must also know your own value. Treat your over-delivery with the care and consideration it deserves. If you are flip about it, they will sense that too, and it will have little value.

About value...

There is *real* value, and there is *perceived* value. When you are booked up and running back to back appointments and your client knows it, those few extra minutes really mean a lot to them. Even if you finished your program with them two minutes earlier and took those two minutes to spend with them, listening and answering questions, they will perceive it as quality time with you and will feel they got more than they paid for.

That feeling of getting more than they paid for is the result of "over-delivering" to your personal training clients.

When you over-deliver, you build excellent clients who are free with referrals and testimonials - the elements you need to grow your business. They become welcome clients, the ones you look forward to working with.

And the foundation of it all?

Relationships.

32

LIPSTICK, PERSONAL TRAINING, AND A SLOWING ECONOMY

Okay, I know what you're thinking…what do lipstick and personal training have in common, and what in the world do they have to do with a slowing economy? Bear with me, and I'll get to that in just a minute.

First of all, let me start by saying that I'm no economist, and I won't even begin to tell you that I understand what's going on with all these crazy bailouts from our leaders in Washington…in fact, I'm not convinced that they even know what's going on, or how to fix the problems. All I can do, with any certainty, is to tell you about my personal experience with slow economic times, and its effect on my personal training business, since the mid 1980's.

I do a lot of consulting work with personal trainers. Recently, there's been a disturbing trend developing. Nearly every trainer I talk with tells me how scared he or she are about these uncertain economic times and they're afraid that the recession will affect their business in a negative way. It's almost like they're giving up before they even get started or they're living a self-fulfilling prophecy where their prediction directly or indirectly causes itself to become true.

My recommendation to these trainers is to look at this as an opportunity, not a death sentence. What I have always observed is that trainers that are willing to get out and hustle are the ones that are the most successful...in good times and bad.

Now, back to the title of this article...Lipstick, Personal Training, and a Slowing Economy. Personal trainers are part of the look good, feel good industry, and when economic times get tough, people look for ways to comfort themselves. There's even something called 'The Lipstick Effect', a phrase coined by Leonard Lauder, retired chairman and heir to the personal products giant, Estee Lauder. It is an economic indicator that some believe is a predictor of slowing economic times. The theory was first identified in the Great Depression, when industrial production in the US fell by half, but sales of cosmetics *rose* between 1929 and 1933. The theory is that *people are willing to spend their money on things that make them look and feel better about themselves*, even when money is tight.

Now, I wasn't around during the Great Depression, but I can give you some historical perspective, specific to the personal training industry, since 1986. In fact, on Monday, October 19, 1987, the stock market lost 22.6% of its total value. To this day, it's still the single largest one-day percentage decline of the DJIA in history. My personal training business was just a little over one year old at the time, and I'll admit that I was nervous. But, by the end of 1987, my personal training business had doubled its revenue from 1986, and doubled again by the end of 1988.

Since I began my business, we've (technically) had three recessions (1990 – 1991, 2001 – 2003, and the most recent one in 2008 – 2009).

From 1990 to 1991, during a recession, cosmetics sales climbed 10%, and my personal training business actually exploded with new clients. The news media kept telling us that the sky was falling...I think the anchor's name was Chicken Little, or something like that. My business had its best two years up to that point in its history, because I chose not to participate in their recession.

Between 2001 and 2003, during another recession, lipstick sales increased by 11% and overall make-up purchases increased as much as 23%. My personal training business actually increased by 25%. Once again, the media told us that the sky was falling, but I chose not to participate.

The recession that began in 2008 has been called the worst recession since the Great Depression. The economy shrank in five quarters, including four quarters in a row. That year my business had its best year ever and followed it up by having even better years in 2009, 2010, and 2011.

In these uncertain times, we have two options...the first option is to accept what the media tells us and wait for our leaders in Washington to make things better (yes I'm being sarcastic), or you can do like I have done and increase your projections for the upcoming year. That's right, I've actually increased my projections and budget each year since 2008 even during economic uncertainty.

So, here's an open invitation to everyone reading this to join me for the good times, and let someone else participate in their recession.

33

7 WAYS TO IMPROVE YOUR MIND/BODY EXPERIENCE

The phrase *mind/body* has been used most often regarding traditional Eastern exercise methods, such as Yoga, Tai Chi, and Qi Gong. These exercise methods incorporate deliberate body movement with meditative and conscious breath work components. They highlight alignment, energy flow, inner awareness, balance, flexibility, and more.

Researchers have discovered many amazing things about mind/body health and healing. While there is still much to learn about this subject, your mind and body have a relationship with each other that is unique to only you. As with all relationships, you can experience growth, friendship, arguments and distance.

According to mindfulness coach and psychologist, Maria Hunt, "we are more likely to achieve our life-enhancing wellness goals when we develop a cooperative relationship between our mind and body and their sometimes-conflicting needs, one that cultivates Focus and Fitness."

Our whole life is intertwined with our very being. Though work, family, and social life may seem separate when viewed from a distance, they are all a very real and immediate part of us and our lifestyle. They provide us with our environments, interactive relationships of give and take, a sense of purpose, fulfillment, stresses, time constraints and deadlines, love and friendship, disagreements, and everything else that is our life.

1. Become aware of your thoughts and words. Are they limiting you? Or are they serving you?

There is one foundational secret to success in achieving breakthroughs: Your brain won't make you a liar. It will align your thoughts & speech to help your body produce exactly what you thought and spoke.

Let me show you this concept in action.

My son, David, and I work out regularly together. I asked him one day how many times he could flip a 300 lb. tractor tire. He thought about it and said, "Four". David is an athlete, strong and quite capable. He flipped the tire four times and was spent, both physically and emotionally.

The next time we worked out, David decided he didn't know how many times he could flip a tire. When he lifted the restrictions he placed on himself, he flipped the tire many more times. David Justice is now unstoppable, because he expanded his thinking and allowed his mind/body relationship to grow with the simple words, "I don't know. Let's see what I can do!"

Your mind/body bottom line: You don't know what you are capable of until you try. Listen to your thoughts and words and adjust them by making them playfully open-ended. What we think and speak becomes our reality. Your mind/body relationship will help you or hinder you in your quest for a Total Body Breakthrough.

Becoming aware of your thinking and speaking will help you to build a better relationship between your mind and body.

2. Know Who You Are

Who are you? We are not static beings. We have experiences every day that we are alive. We can be whoever and do whatever we want at any given time, with few exceptions.

What are your beliefs about your body, your health, "acting your age", your capabilities, your needs and desires, food, time, money, freedom? Have you bought into the myths of "old age"?

Do you have a list of things you are not "good" at?

Your identity is who you believe yourself to be. You may have accepted someone else's perspective of you, never questioned it, and adopted it as your own. Perhaps someone told you often when you were younger that you were no good at sports, and you spent your life believing this, never attempting any physical activities. Or perhaps you came up with an interpretation on your own, such as when you noticed that you had to "work" at something that came easily to someone else – by being "a comparing creature," in other words.

Is your identity tied to your weight, a disability, a perceived weakness, your body shape, your expertise, your job, your sport, your family, your personality, your smile, or your hair color?

What would happen to your identity if any of those factors change? If you have tied your identity to something that no longer is, you may feel you no longer know who you are. You are who you are or who you let others (or your own unbalanced beliefs) dictate who you are (which limits what you can do and become).

Your mind/body bottom line: You are not your weight; you are not your medals and diplomas. Those are what you look like and what you've done. You are not the same person you were last year. You have retained some of your foundational beliefs. Are they helping or hurting you? Which ones do you want to feed?

3. Listen to Your Body

Your body talks to you in many different ways. From the moment you awaken until you fall asleep, it speaks to you with emotion, physical sensations, memories, and urges to action (or inaction).

If you are carrying excess weight on your body, your knees (designed for your average size body) are now being taxed with excessive force and being made to move under duress. They creak and groan, they complain and protest as their cartilage and surface structures wear away under that pressure and strain. They send pain signals through your body to your mind, screaming, STOP!

You can choose to sit and limit your movement because your knees hurt or you can choose to lose the weight your knees are complaining about.

A client with a shoulder that was pretty much immobile acknowledged holding her purse on the right for most of her life (she's in her mid 80s), and then years later replaced her purse with a cane in that hand. Continued unconscious "holding" of her arm ensured that the muscles, joints, and tendons would also stay immobile. After weeks of exercise her shoulder was freed up. She had to relearn how to move the arm without shrugging her shoulder, and lose the tendency to "protect" it.

Become aware of what your body is telling you.

You can compensate for it or you can do something that will create a more natural, pleasing, and long lasting result for you.

Your mind/body bottom line: What is your body saying to you? Are you listening to it? Are you responding proactively?

4. Pay Attention to Your Own Experience, Your Own Reality, This Very Moment.

Eleanor Roosevelt once said, "No one can make you feel inferior without your consent." You may not be able to control the experience of your emotions in the moment, but you can explore your feelings or bring another emotion to the forefront of your awareness.

I had a client who broke her arm in 35 places and her doctor told her she would never regain full use of that arm. I disagreed. She could have taken the doctor at his word and simply given up. She chose instead to work with me and now has full use of her arm.

Nothing in life is ever as it was. Time and circumstances change everything, sometimes for the better, sometimes not. We can embrace this moment or cling to the past, move forward, or surrender.

You wouldn't drive a car with your eyes closed. When you walk down an icy, snow covered slope, or use power tools, where is your focus? Lost in the joy of a hobby or activity you love, time just flies by. Your focus and concentration is on the task at hand. When we focus on something we make progress, we learn, we get somewhere.

Whatever we do consistently is called practice or habit. Repetition is how we learned to write, ride a bike, drive, play a sport, and all the other things we do well or regularly. Practice is a conscious effort at duplicating something. Habit is an unconscious action that once served a purpose for us that may or may not produce the same benefit we felt when we started it. Turning the light off when you leave a room is a habit that still serves a purpose.

The more we sit on a couch, the better we get at it. The more we go outside and play, the better we get at it. The more we listen to our words, our bodies, and our thoughts, the better we get at it.

Your mind/body bottom line: Become aware of what you are "practicing". It will become a part of your lifestyle very fast. Line up your thoughts, words, and actions with your objectives for your Total Body Breakthrough and things will fall into place for you more quickly.

5. The Inevitable Consequences of Action and Inaction

Your body has specific needs to regain and retain its health. You as a person have specific needs that nurture your mental, emotional, and physical health.

Developing your mind/body relationship will help you bring balance to your plan of action, and savor the moments that will bring you closer to your desires.

If you do not give your body the fresh air, sunshine, water, regular exercise, proper nutrition, sleep, and stress reduction it needs to stay healthy, your health will deteriorate. A fresh egg, dropped on a concrete floor, will break. If we don't proactively make healthy choices for our body, our body will decide our health status for us based on the tools we give it, or don't.

There are so many types of exercise and so many different flavors and textures of natural, healthy food available. Explore them, you WILL find something you like and will stick with.

Whichever exercise method you choose, your body will respond. Regular exercise and proper nutrition will be your friend, if you let them.

Your mind/body bottom line: Find the healthy lifestyle activities that work for you and do them. When you find what works for you, you will stick with it. You can easily make time for things you love in your life – making time for health is easier when you discover the methods you enjoy.

6. Where is Your Finish Line?

Margie participated in a transformation program and succeeded in looking great for her wedding, then life got busy, and the kids came. 12 years, 47 lbs. and 2 daily prescriptions later, Margie decided to do another transformation program. Her plan: this program would be her jump-start to regain her health and set her on track to a lifetime of good health.

For a future Olympian, the finish line is the gold medal podium, not simply getting to the Olympics, or being first at the finish line. It is standing on that podium with gold medal held high and that rush of recognition that they are the best in the world.

For many of us who are not world-class athletes, the finish line is the end of a long, healthy, and prosperous life, free of disability and chronic illness with all of our faculties intact. For others, it's the class reunion or a family wedding to get into shape for, with no thought for the years to follow.

Health and fitness is a lifelong journey. One tank of gas will only get you as far as one tank of gas. Likewise, you must provide your body with proper nutrition and regular exercise as part of your everyday life for the rest of your life in order to see continued health and fitness benefits.

Your mind/body bottom line: How far out is your finish line? Is this Total Body Breakthrough a jump-start to the next mile marker? When we are a work in progress and have something to strive for, our mind/body relationship tends to cooperate for success.

7. Does Your Reality Support Your Possibilities?

Your Mind/Body relationship grows or stagnates through your thoughts, words, and actions. Your identity is tightly woven into your mind and body.

The key to refining your reality is to discover what you truly want, enjoy and will stick with, knowing where your finish line is, and knowing that you are capable of more. A vibrant and healthy reality is there for you, should you choose to accept it.

When you practice healthy lifestyles, you will become healthier. When you practice thinking with possibilities, almost all things become possible. When you speak hopefully, positively, and confidently, your posture, stature, and thinking becomes empowering.

Grab hold of the very basic truths in this book and find a way to make them work for you.

- Write down your objectives, keep them visible. Journal so you can see how you are progressing.

- Make the time for the activities you know will help you get where you want to go, schedule them.

- Very few of us are self-motivated in every area of our lives. Find that buddy who will help hold you accountable to your plan of action, encourage you, support and celebrate your achievements, no matter how small.

Your mind/body bottom line: You have a natural mind/body relationship that can help you succeed in your Total Body Breakthrough. Work with it, stay with it.

You can learn to be your own best friend and use your mind/body experience to achieve more of what you want.

Make a difference in your mind, and you'll make a difference in your body.

34

UNITED WE STAND…
AGAINST OUR COMMON ENEMY

…THE PRETENDERS AMONG US

(They are in your backyard and are eating out of your future)

The Pretenders have usurped our profession for the last time…

WARNING: The Information You Are about to Read is ONLY For Those Personal Trainers Who Believe that the World's Newest Profession has been Tainted and Flouted Like it Were the Oldest and Want to Take Back Their Integrity and Worth.

First, I'd like to tell you a story that I hope will inspire you.

I love all of my clients, yet one market is especially near and dear to my heart. Corporate accounts. Working as a business owner with other business owners in pursuit of a common goal – employee wellness and productivity – has been very rewarding for me.

One day I was online reading some results of a variety of corporate wellness programs. One of the studies that touted its program as a success was one where they had placed every employee with high cholesterol on medication to bring the cholesterol level back in range. There was no fitness program in place. There was no nutrition program in place.

I felt outrage that a "doctor" who took an oath to "first do no harm" would even consider managing disease instead of first applying healthy measures such as suggesting a change in diet and implementing a regular exercise program.

Don't get me wrong. I know there is a time and a place for disease management. There are some unreasonable people out there and equally as many people who don't want to take responsibility for themselves, their own actions and the resulting consequences. These are the most difficult clients we have, if we can even get them as clients in the first place.

We simply MUST get to the root of any problem to effectively address a solution. If we look only to the symptoms of a thing and not expose the root of that problem, we are only offering a band-aid solution. Addressing the root cause will help to generate effective and more permanent solutions.

The whole issue of Health Care Reform is so loaded with widely differing views on each side of the fence that even professionals can't agree on major points, much less the entire scope of it.

I was writing rants (in my humble, yet very direct way) to some of the blogs and editorials that I was reading. As I was raging against supposedly "professional", "educated", and "knowledgeable experts" my brain suddenly replayed many of my clients' faces.

I was re-visiting their agony and pain as they recounted to me the horror stories of unprofessional behavior from their previous personal trainer. Their experiences ranged from receiving inappropriate comments to incompetent training methods and varying degrees of poor and unprofessional behavior.

It made me uncomfortable to hear about the unprofessional conduct of some people claiming the title and rank of personal trainer, my profession, when they had little more than a high school diploma and a weekend certification course.

Trainers who exercise their clients' way beyond the client's capabilities, do little to minimize injury, or taunt and demoralize their clients are way more common than I used to think. What happens to those clients when that unprofessional and incompetent trainer loses them? Some are turned off forever from the very thought of exercising. Some showed up at my door. I'm sure some showed up at your door, willing to give it another shot.

Rebuilding trust is not an easy matter. For an entire industry to have an identity problem because of the scattered, unprofessional, and incompetent trainers – The Pretenders – is unthinkable.

Identity Theft?

No. We gave it away, and maybe we never had our own identity to begin with.

The concept of Personal Training is lumped in with gym rat, group instructor, recreation and activity director.

I believe that one reason our industry has an identity problem is because we have not properly identified ourselves to each other and to the world, the exercising and not-yet-exercising public.

Who Needs a Personal Trainer?

Another reason is perception of the public about workouts. Even we encourage people to workout in between their workouts with us, and that perception is they don't need us all the time, that they are competent to workout on their own. There are government recommendations about the number of and amount of time for workouts to achieve positive health benefits. Those recommendations are for everyone with a body.

The perception of self-help, quick fix, magic pill, and exercise paraphernalia that is marketed through hype and infomercials has flooded the consumer mind with misinformation, hope of achievement without much action on their part, and discouragement as they try to find their way alone through that confusing maze.

Personal Trainers Need Personal Trainers Now, More Than Ever.

We need to stand up united, lifting our voices together to maintain the ethical integrity and professional standing of the Personal Trainer.

The Pretenders among us are undermining your determination, drive, and ambition for your business and your lifestyle. You have worked too hard to lose any of what you have gained.

The lack of standardized requirements to enter our industry as a qualified professional allows the Pretenders to have free reign in YOUR market, bouncing in and out of the Scope of Practice of the Personal Trainer, allowing them to instruct by personal opinion...a very dangerous proposition to say the least. This ability they have simply undermines and drags down the professional and ethical integrity of our profession and puts the public at risk.

Perhaps you, too, are awed at the concept of helping people regain and retain their health, to look good and feel great. I can't think of a more enjoyable way to spend my days. Yet, we hold their safety in our hands. One wrong decision, one lax judgment on my part could cause serious injury to my client.

We also hold in our hands their motivation, desire, and dreams to reinforce or destroy. That is a privilege that I take very seriously, as I am sure you do.

The Pretenders are a Cancer...

...that must be cut out at the root.

They will be made to stand up and be accountable through the tireless efforts of trainers like you and me to promote professionalism in the marketplace and a positive image among consumers.

FINAL THOUGHTS

I hope you've enjoyed some of my stories, advice and experiences during my first 30 years in the personal training industry...lot's more to come.

When I started my career in the early 80's, there weren't any Gurus, with done-for-you systems. We were pretty much on our own, trying to figure things out. Fortunately, I was born with pig-headed determination (my wife calls it being "stubborn"), and I wasn't going to accept being told; "This will never work in Kansas City. You'll have to move to New York or L.A., because Kansas City is way too conservative to support a business like yours." That's what a legendary Kansas City radio broadcaster told me during my first live interview in August of 1986. He sat about three feet from me, blowing cigar smoke in my direction and telling the entire city that my business would fail.

Needless to say, I didn't let his words squash my dreams. To quote a long-time client, Henry Bloch, from his book "Many Happy Returns, "Don't bet against the underdog who refuses to quit." Persistence, determination and focus will prevail almost every time.

These days, trainers have an incredible advantage with done-for-you business, marketing, and workout protocol products and services. There are mastermind groups and franchise opportunities that hold trainers accountable and keep them on the cutting edge of an ever-changing industry.

There are so many incredible groups, organizations, blogs and industry publications, but only so much time in a day. I know this isn't a complete list and there are many that I'm leaving out, but the ones I've listed are some of my favorites.

Blogs I read and/or contribute to:
Brian Grasso – FreeThinkingRenegade.com
Chris McCombs – KickBackLife.com
Curtis Mock – FitBiz.tv
Dave Schmitz – ResistanceBandTraining.com
EricCressey.com
Erik Rokeach – FitnessBusinessInterviews.com
FitBusinessInsider.com
FitnessMarketingMuscle.com
JohnSpencerEllis.com
Mike Robertson – RobertsonTrainingSystems.com
Sam Bakhtiar – Super-Trainer.com
Underground Strength Training – ZachEven-esh.com

Publications I read and/or contribute to:
Personal Fitness Professional magazine (PFP)
IDEA Fitness Journal
Club Industry magazine
Club Solutions
Personal Trainer Today

My websites and contact information:
AYCFit.com
GregJustice.com
KansasCityPersonalTrainer.com
CorporateBootCampSystem.com
info@aycfit.com

I NEED YOUR HELP!

I've shared with you some of my favorite stories. Now I'd love to hear some of yours.

My next project is a compilation of stories, advice, and anecdotes from personal trainers around the world that will inform, educate, and inspire others to continue the art of making a difference in people's lives.

Your submissions can be funny, serious, heartwarming, useful, inspirational, personal…you get the idea. Just be sincere, truthful, and willing to share stories that have helped you become a better person and trainer.

Tell me how you handled the situation and, if you could do it all over again, how you may have done it differently.

Submit your stories to me at:

info@aycfit.com

Thanks!
Greg

ABOUT THE AUTHOR

GREG JUSTICE, MA

"Training veteran Greg Justice didn't just get in on the leading edge of an emerging industry, he helped create it. Opening the first personal training studio in Kansas City, Justice has, over the years, laid the groundwork for countless others to follow.

Being a trailblazer, however, takes a willingness to plow into the thicket of uncertainty. It means forging ahead with nothing but faith. As one of the true leaders of the personal training industry, Justice now has the benefit of hindsight and the insight of experience, both of which he eagerly offers up to the hundreds of trainers he has mentored."

– Shelby Murphy, Editor, Personal
Fitness Professional magazine

Greg Justice, is an international best-selling author, speaker and fitness entrepreneur.

He opened **AYC Health & Fitness**, Kansas City's Original Personal Training Center, in May 1986, and has personally trained more than 46,000 one-on-one sessions. Today, AYC specializes in corporate wellness as well as personal training.

Greg holds a master's degree in HPER (exercise science) (1986) from Morehead State University, Morehead, KY and a bachelor's degree in Health & Physical Education (1983) from Morehead State University, Morehead, KY.

He has worked with athletes and non-athletes of all ages and physical abilities and served as a conditioning coach at the collegiate level. He also worked with the Kansas City Chiefs, during the offseason, in the early 1980's.

He has been actively involved in the fitness industry for more than a quarter of a century as a club manager, owner, personal fitness trainer, and corporate wellness supervisor where he worked with more than 64 corporations. Greg writes articles for many international publications and websites including Exercise & Health, IDEA Fitness Journal, American Fitness Magazine, Protraineronline.com, Fitcommerce.com, is a featured columnist for Corporate Wellness Magazine, and has a monthly column called "Treadmill Talks" in Personal Fitness Professional (PFP) magazine. He has authored books titled "Lies & Myths about Corporate Wellness", "Treadside Manner – Confessions of a Serial Personal Trainer" and was a contributing author for two other books.

Greg served as an adjunct professor of exercise science at Avila University and currently serves on the advisory board of two personal training schools. He mentors and instructs trainers interested in Personal Training and Corporate Wellness through his Coaching Programs and Corporate Boot Camp System class, which spans nine countries, 45 states and six Canadian Provinces.